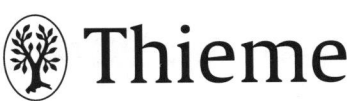

Fachenglisch für Pflegeberufe

Brush up your English – fast and easy

Ank van de Wiel

Unter Mitarbeit von Gabriela Schmitz
(Unit 11 Nursing process)

Deutsche Übersetzung von
Gerhard Uppenbrink

2., überarbeitete Auflage

Georg Thieme Verlag
Stuttgart · New York

Titel der holländischen Originalausgabe:
Engels voor verpleegkundigen
en andere werkers in de gezondheidszorg
© Bohn Stafleu van Loghum bv, Houten, 1996
Alle Rechte vorbehalten

Übersetzung:
Übersetzungsdienst Uppenbrink
Postfach 1463
D-70810 Korntal-Münchingen

Die Deutsche Bibliothek – CIP-Einheitsaufnahme

Wiel, Ank van de:
Fachenglisch für Pflegeberufe / Ank van de Wiel.
Dt. Übers. von Gerhard Uppenbrink.
2. Aufl. - Stuttgart : Thieme, 2002
 Einheitssacht.: Engels voor verpleegkundigen en andere
 werkers in de gezondheidsorg <dt.>

1. Auflage 1998

© 1998, 2002 Georg Thieme Verlag,
Rüdigerstraße 14,
D-70469 Stuttgart
Unsere Homepage: http://www.thieme.de

Printed in Germany

ISBN 3-13-115062-9   1 2 3 4 5 6

Vorwort

Ihnen liegt die revidierte Version des Leitfadens **„Fachenglisch für Pflegeberufe"** vor. Ich freue mich, dass so viele Menschen von der ersten Ausgabe Gebrauch gemacht haben und ich hoffe, dass dies erneut der Fall sein wird. Eine Anzahl von Texten ist durch mehr aktuelle Versionen ersetzt worden. Des Weiteren ist das Buch um einige Sprachfertigkeitsübungen und um Original-Berichtsmaterial ergänzt worden. Die Praxis zeigt immer noch, dass Studenten und andere Benutzer dieses Buches als eine Kombination von Lernen und Üben schätzen.

Ich bin den Studenten der Hochschulen Arnhem und Nijmegen wiederum für deren Beitrag an der Neufassung des Buches dankbar. Die Themen im Buch sind ausgerichtet auf die allgemeine Gesundheitsfürsorge, da die meisten Pflegeberufe sich im Ausland dafür entscheiden. Das Buch ist nicht dazu bestimmt, die pflegerischen oder medizinischen Kenntnisse zu testen, sondern um Sprachfertigkeit in Englisch zu erweitern, zu erproben und zu üben.

Jeder Abschnitt hat **ein** Hauptthema, an das alle Übungen im Abschnitt anschließen. Das Buch ist sowohl für die klassische Verwendung als auch für Selbststudien geeignet. Im Prinzip wird die britische Orthographie verwendet. Im hinteren Teil des Buches finden Sie eine Vokabelsammlung. Die Übersetzung der Vokabeln bezieht sich ausschließlich auf den gegebenen Kontext.

Ich möchte mich auch bei Drs. Wilma Lamers für ihre Empfehlungen bezüglich der Grammatik bedanken. Bemerkungen oder Ergänzungen zum Leitfaden sind mehr als willkommen.

Nijmegen,
Ank van de Wiel

Inhaltsverzeichnis

Medical Personnel

1.1 Health Care in Britain and the US

Text

Undoubtedly, the characteristic that most distinguishes between the health systems of the UK and the US is the extent and nature of governmental involvement in financing, regulating and providing health services. In both countries governmental involvement in health has been evolutionary. Government's earliest assumption of responsibility came in the field of public health – the control of the spread of infectious diseases. Governmental involvement in the provision of health services to individuals is a recent phenomenon. Earlier health care had been offered mainly as private enterprises. Health care was considered an item of personal consumption – like a loaf of bread – to be bought and paid for by the individual consumer on a fee-for-service basis. Health facilities were mostly privately owned. Health care providers, to the extent that they were formally trained, received their educations without government support. The notion that provision of health care to individuals is a public responsibility is attributed to Otto von Bismarck (Roemer, 1985). An army survey had found Germany's youth to be appalingly unfit for military service, and as Germany maintained a large army, the health of the nation's youth had to be improved. In 1883 the German chancellor also promoted the adoption of compulsory health insurance for industrial workers to receive medical treatment so that they might return to productive employment sooner. From the 1920s onwards, compulsory health insurance in Germany was gradually expanded to all segments of society. Interestingly although the UK was industrially more advanced than Germany, it did not adopt a governmentally mandated health insurance system until 1911. In that year the National Health Insurance Act created compulsory health insurance programme for low income workers that provided coverage for services of a general practitioner (GP). As a result of the National Health Service Act of 1946, the National Health Service established in 1948 effected sweeping changes in the organization and delivery of health care. Financed largely by general taxation, insurance benefits were extended to the entire population to include free hospitalization (hospitals had become part of the NHS) and dental, ophthalmic, home nursing and other services. In the US some forms of voluntary health insurance programmes had existed since the beginning of the twentieth century, including workmen's compensation programmes and sickness funds administered by beneficial societies. Commercial health insurance was a rarity until the advent of the Blue Cross plan for hospital insurance (initiated in 1929). It was supplemented in the 1930s by the Blue Shield programme of coverage for medical services. These programmes grew to be major suppliers of health insurance. Today private health insurance in the US finances about a third of total personal health care expenditure (Levitt, 1985). The only national health insurance system is Medicare for people 65 years of age and over. In 1973 disabled persons, their dependents and those with end-stage renal disease were added to the scheme. Expenditure for Medicare in 1989 comprised over 20% of total US health expenditure. Thus the governmental role in the health systems of the two countries has evolved quite differently. The British NHS, financed largely by general taxation and providing essentially free care, is the system with the most government control. The American health 'system' is described as pluralistic, mixed or segmented leaving 30 to 36 million people with no health insurance.

Bron: Nursing practice in the UK and North America, Chapman & Hall

Answer the following questions about the text.

1. *distinguishes in line 2 means*:
   a) resembles
   b) differentiates
   c) stimulates
   d) protects

2. *involvement in line 7 means*:
   a) resistance
   b) knowledge
   c) help
   d) participation

3. *provision in line 12 means*:
   a) supply
   b) support
   c) provocation
   d) protection

4. *responsibility in line 25 refers to*:
   a) care
   b) concern
   c) service
   d) accountability

5. *appalingly in line 27 means*:
   a) horribly
   b) splendidly
   c) increasingly
   d) unfortunately

6. *compulsory in line 32 means*:
   a) optionally
   b) required by law
   c) deliberately
   d) free

7. *Act in line 43 means*:
   a) policy
   b) a written order of a parliament
   c) suggestion
   d) behaviour

8. *GP in line 47 means*:
   a) pharmacist
   b) dentist
   c) consultant
   d) a doctor working in the community

9. *funds in line 61 means*:
   a) insurances
   b) benefits
   c) money resources
   d) regulations

10. *health insurance in line 62 means*:
    a) a contract of insurance concerning health care
    b) a guarantee to be healthy
    c) a payment for health
    d) reassurance

1.2 Nurses

Conversation There are many different kinds of medical personnel, including doctors, nurses, physiotherapists and medical scientists. They all have a specific job to do. Medical scientists, for example, analyse samples and research new techniques for treating illness. A physiotherapist helps people to move properly after an illness or accident. Doctors and nurses look after patients in different areas of medicine. We will concentrate on nursing first.

Jenny, Mike and *Jill* are all nurses. They do, however, work in different areas or fields of nursing. Listen to the conversation they have with an interviewer *(I)*.

I: Hello! Which one of you works in a hospital?

Jenny: Well, we all work in a kind of hospital, but there are different names for it.

Mike: That's right. Jenny works in a *general hospital,* Jill works in an *institution for the mentally handicapped* and I work in a *psychiatric* [ˌsaɪkɪˈætrɪk] *hospital* or *mental clinic.*

I: Have you ever worked with Jenny or Mike?

Jill: Yes, I have actually, when I was carrying out one of my placements as a student nurse. During our training we have to work for a short period in other fields of nursing. At one time we all worked in a geriatric ward of a general hospital. That was real good fun because we enjoy working together. I think it is very useful to work in all areas before you finish your training. It broadens your scope a little.

I: So, what are your qualifications now, are they different from the other two?

Jenny: Oh yes, we have a different registration. Mike is an **RMN,** which stands for *registered mental nurse,* and Jill is an **RNMH,** which refers to *registered nurse for the mentally handicapped,* and I am an **RGN,** a *registered general nurse* or **RN** as they call it in the USA.

I: What is the main difference between your job and, let's say, Jenny's?

Mike: Well, Jenny deals mostly with people who suffer from physical problems and I work with people who have mental problems. Although sometimes people suffer from both. It is not always easy to separate the two.

I: And what about your patients?

Jill: A nurse for the mentally handicapped looks after people who cannot be independent because of a congenital mental deficiency. Although the cause of the illness is physical we have to deal with a lot of psychological problems as well.

I: Do all your colleagues have the same qualifications?

Jenny: No, they don't. Most teams, in all three areas, work with nurses and helpers with different grades and qualifications, for example: **ENS** or *enrolled nurses* and **NA/ANS** or *nursing assistants/ancillary nurses.*

I: So many different names for the same job?

Jill: Well, it is not exactly the same job. Every worker has specific tasks according to his or her qualification or grade. It is the same team but it can be a completely different job.

I: Well, thank you all very much for your time.

All: You're welcome.

Exercise   Translate the following words from the conversation.

1. _____ Laborant

2. _____ Ausbildung

3. _____ Psychiatrische Einrichtung

4. _____ Fortbildung

5. _____ Diplome

6. _____ trennen

7. _____ psychische Probleme

8. _____ angeboren

9. _____ Pflegehilfe

10. _____ Niveau

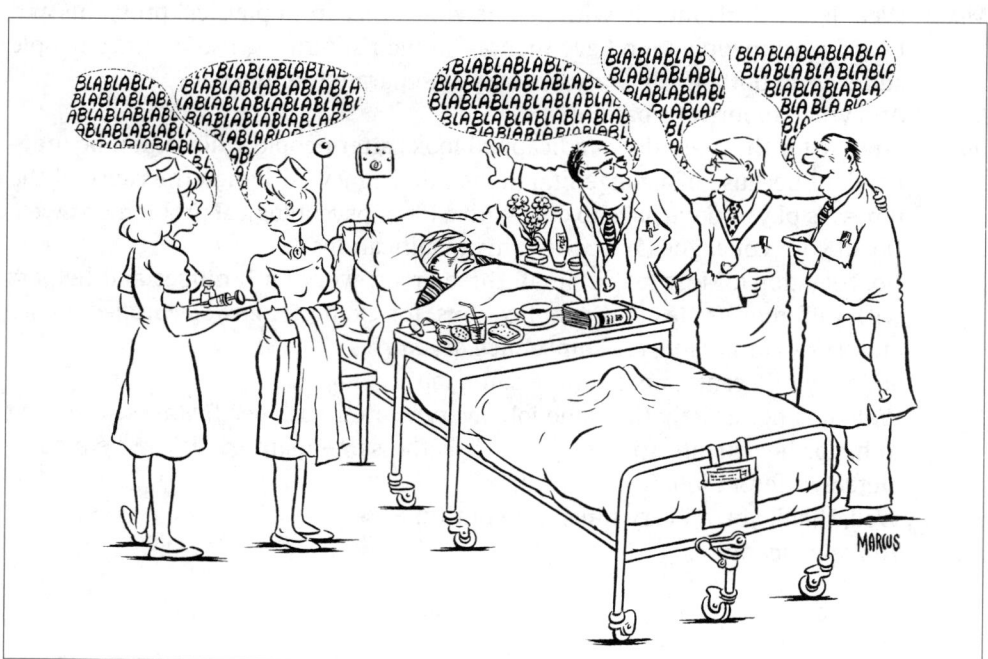

Quelle: Löwensteiner Cartoon Service (Hrsg.): Dr. med. Ironicus. Thieme, Stuttgart 1994 (S. 75)

1.3 Nursing Qualifications

Specific area		Information
general nursing		A-Pflege
RGN	registered general nurse	A-Pfleger/in
mental nursing		B-Pflege
RMN	registered mental nurse	B-Pfleger/in
mentally handicapped nursing		Z-Pflege
RNMH	registered nurse for the mentally handicapped	Z-Pfleger/in
paediatric nursing		Kinderpflege
RSCN	registered sick children's nurse	Kinderpfleger/in

All areas		
EN (UK)	enrolled nurse	Pfleger/in 2. Grades
LPN (USA)	licensed practical nurse	Krankenhelfer/in
LVN (USA)	licensed vocational nurse	Krankenhelfer/in
NA (UK + USA)	nursing assistant	Pflegehilfe
AN (UK + USA)	ancillary nurse	Pflegehilfe

BN: bachelor of nursing
DN: diploma of nursing

Britsh Grades:

Grade C: enrolled or auxiliary nurse
Grade D: newly qualified nurse
Grade E: experienced staff nurse
Grade F: senior nurse
Grade G: sister/charge nurse
Grade H: nurse specialist
Grade I: nurse specialist
Nurse consultant

1.4 The Medical Team

Nurses usually work shifts to run hospital wards 24 hours a day. They are assisted by student nurses, in addition to the nurses already mentioned. The nurse who is in charge of the ward is called *sister* (when female) or *charge nurse* (male or female). Many ancillary, or supportive, departments are needed to provide the service in the patient care units.

Exercise

Where do you go when:

1. a doctor sends your patient for an MRI investigation?
2. your patient needs to improve his cooking skills?
3. your pay-check is incorrect?
4. the bell push from one of your patients does not work?
5. a patient cannot go home due to lack of family support?
6. a urine specimen needs to be tested?
7. your patient wants his diet changed?
8. a patient cannot communicate well due to aphasia?
9. your patient needs to learn how to walk again?
10. you need medication that your ward does not have in stock?
11. the standard of hygiene in a room is not as it should be?

... **a)** *Business services department:* takes care of financial matters.
... **b)** *Dietary department:* provides meals for patients and staff.
... **c)** *Housekeeping department/domestics:* clean the hospital.
... **d)** *Maintenance service department:* cares for and repairs equipment.
... **e)** *Physiotherapy department:* uses physical methods to promote healing, including the use of light, heat, electric current, massage, manipulation and remedial exercise.
... **f)** *Occupational therapy department:* helps people to reach their maximum level of function and independence in all aspects of life.
... **g)** *Pathology department:* examines body tissues and fluids and carries out laboratory tests.
... **h)** *Pharmacy department:* prepares and dispenses medication.
... **i)** *Radiology/X-ray department:* takes X-rays and uses radioactive substances in the diagnosis and treatment of diseases.
... **j)** *Social services department:* provides counselling, financial advice and sometimes arranges transfers.
... **k)** *Speech therapy department:* helps patients to speak and communicate more effectively after loss of this ability.

Do you know any other departments or people you work with?

1.5 Health Care in the USA

Text

1 The USA provides for medical service in a different way than Great Britain does. Social security schemes including health care are: Medicare, Medicaid, Workmen's 5 compensation, Maternal and child health services, Indian health service, Veteran's hospital and medical care. Of these, Medicare and Medicaid are the largest ones. Medicare is a national (federal) in- 10 surance which mainly covers the expenses for health care for people of 65 years and older and for handicapped people who have been on an invalidity benefit for over two years.

15 Medicaid was primarily started to support people who were receiving benefits through the Social Security Act, but this was soon extended to all people of limited means. Its aim was to put an end to a 20 health care which was (until then) large- ly financed by charitable agencies. Besides these schemes the cost of health care is met by private and group insurance plans and expenditures directly paid 25 by patients. Although there were discussions to have a health system similar to that of the UK, concern about rising costs prevented adoption of a national insurance system.

30 Health care expenditure has risen to 12% of the gross national product, which is the highest percentage in the world. Nevertheless, the efficacy and equity of these costs are questionable since a high pro- 35 portion of Americans are dissatisfied with the system. Cause for concern are the 30 million people in the USA without a health insurance. In the years ahead, access to health care might become a privi- 40 lege to the lucky or wealthy few.

Fluency: How to give advice

Exercise

When you give advice it is helpful when:

- you tune your advice to your patient's/client's need;
- you know how well your patient/client can process the information;
- you are familiar with your patient's/client's social environment;
- you are familiar with your patient's/client's living and working situation;
- you are informed of the advice and treatment given so far.

Phrases that can be used by nurses:

- What seems to be the problem sir/madam?
- How long have you been suffering from this problem?
- Does it hurt?
- When does it hurt?
- What sort of treatment have you tried before?
- Do you have any other complaints?

Phrases that are used by patients/clients:

- I don't feel very well.
- I have been very ill since ...
- I have a terrible pain in ...
- My child doesn't want to ...
- I have been suffering from ...
- I can't use my ...
- My medication doesn't work/is out of date/is finished ...
- I don't know how to ...

Exercise   Now find a partner and practice a conversation between a nurse and a patient/client in the following situations:

1: A nurse receives a phone call from a mother. Her four-year-old child has been admitted with diarrhoea. He does not want to eat and only wants to drink. She is very worried he will dehydrate and wants to know how he is and what you are going to do with him.
   As the nurse you try to reassure her, tell her the child is in good hands and that she can come to the ward any time she wants.

2: A patient wants some advice about different incontinence products.
   As the nurse you discuss the following products: special bedmaterial (covers, sheets and pads, incontinence material; diapers/nappies, plastic pants).

3: A patient tells you that she is pregnant and that she is thinking of cancelling all treatment because she thinks it will harm her baby.
   As the nurse you advise this client to continue her treatment and hat there will be no danger and no x-rays will be taken. Explain also that all medication used is safe.

1.6 The Continuous Tense (Verlaufsform)

Grammar   Die Verlaufsform wird mit „*to be*" + Verb in der „*-ing*-Form" gebildet.

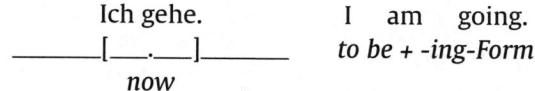

Ich gehe. I am going.
to be + -ing-Form
now

Der Zeitbalken gibt den Moment des Sprechens mit einem Punkt (.) und dem Wörtchen „now" an. Die eckigen Klammern umschließen die Zeit, die die Verbform berührt.

Diese Form gibt an, dass:

1. *etwas im Gange ist und kurz andauert*
   Are you changing the bed?   Machst du gerade das Bett?
   He was dying when we arrived.   Er starb, als wir ankamen.

2. *etwas in naher Zukunft geschehen wird*
   She is coming to our ward tonight.   Sie kommt heute abend in unsere
                                            Abteilung.
   He is having an operation tomorrow.   Er wird morgen operiert.

3. *etwas häufig geschieht und ein negatives Gefühl erzeugt*
   Why are you never helping us?   Warum helfen Sie uns nie?
   She is always complaining about her   Sie beklagt sich ständig über das
   staff.   Personal.

1.7 Translation

Translate the following sentences.   *Exercise*

1. Schreiben Sie an dieses Krankenhaus, wenn Sie eine neue Stelle suchen.

   _____

2. Ich bewerbe mich um die Stelle des Abteilungsleiters.

   _____

3. Über diesen Pflegeanwärter ärgere ich mich sehr.

   _____

4. Der Physiotherapeut übt mit ihm.

   _____

5. Der Logopäde versucht, ihre Kommunikationsfähigkeiten zu verbessern.

   _____

1.8 Prepositions

Use one of the following prepositions to fill in the gaps.   *Exercise*
to   from   at   by   in   with   on   of

1. I am going _____ see the doctor.

2. To take samples _____ the throat.

3. He works _____ St. Mary's Hospital.

4. I usually travel _____ air.

5. Who let him _____ ?

6. The patient made it, you're _____ luck.

7. He had a throbbing pain _____ his side.

8. _____ what I know, he is very ill.

9. I was held up _____ a patient.

10. Who do you work _____ ?

11. I know her _____ sight.

12. I'll go _____ or without you.

13. She's _____ the bathroom.

14. That hospital is _____ the seaside.

15. Eggs are rich _____ protein.

16. The charge nurse is looking for a list _____ names.

17. She was speaking _____ a clear voice.

18. I hand him over _____ you.

19. He missed me _____ an inch.

20. Let's start _____ this room today.

1.9 Specialized Nurses

Exercise

There are many nurses who work in a specialist area. A midwife, for example, is a nurse who is an expert at delivering babies.

See if you can find the right description for the right job.

1. district nurse
2. community psychiatric nurse (CPN)
3. occupational health nurse
4. practice nurse
5. school nurse
6. theatre nurse
7. sick children's nurse (RSCN)
8. A and E nurse
9. IC nurse
10. obstetric nurse

... **a)** Employed by general practitioners (GPS) to work in the treatment room/surgery.

... **b)** A qualified nurse with special training in domiciliary services, assessing, prescribing and evaluating nursing plans for patients in the community.

... **c)** Nurses women during pregnancy, childbirth and the period following the birth.

... **d)** Specially trained nurse who looks after young children usually on paediatric wards of a general hospital.

... **e)** Visits people in their own homes to give advice, assess the mental state of the patient and control medication.

... **f)** Passes instruments to the surgeon and generally assists at the operation.

... **g)** Examines the workplace for accidents/illness, is involved in preventative teaching, medical examination of new workers, maintaining records as well as running a surgery at hours which workers can attend.

... **h)** Specially trained nurse in the health care of school-age children, who is responsible for monitoring growth and development and for screening out the abnormal and who has responsibility for children with special educational needs.

... **i)** Nurse who works in the accident and emergency unit of a hospital where people are brought in after an accident or when they need emergency treatment.

... **j)** Nurse who is trained in specialized and monitored health care for critically ill and immediately postoperative patients in a specially designed unit (IC/CC).

1.10 The (Simple) Present Tense

Das Präsens wird durch das **ganze Verb + „(e)s"** gebildet. *Grammar*
Sie arbeitet in dieser Abteilung

she works in this ward
←------------→ Präsens

Diese Form gibt an, dass:

1. *es um einen Fakt oder eine Tatsache geht*
   She tests her blood sugar level in the morning.   Morgens kontrolliert sie ihren Blutzuckerspiegel.
   This patient lives in the country.   Dieser Patient wohnt auf dem Land.

2. *etwas normal ist oder wiederholt vorkommt*
   We always give the children a hot drink.   Wir geben den Kindern immer etwas Warmes zu trinken
   They usually switch the lights off at 10 pm.   Sie machen meistens um 22.00 Uhr das Licht aus.

3. *etwas im gleichen Moment passiert oder sinngemäß wahrgenommen wird*
   Here she comes.   Dort ist sie.
   Do you hear that alarm?   Hörst du den Alarm?

4. *die Rede von einem festen Schema, einem Programm oder einem Raster ist*
   The operation starts at 8 am.   Die Operation beginnt um 8.00 Uhr morgens.
   My plane leaves at midnight.   Mein Flugzeug geht um 12.00 Uhr nachts.

Choose the correct form.

Exercise

1. This man *is always complaining/always complains*.
2. Water *is freezing/freezes* at zero degrees Celsius.
3. Look! He *bleeds/is bleeding*.
4. June *is leaving/leaves* for India on Monday.
5. Our plane *is arriving/arrives* in Bombay at 10.30.
6. The homehelp *is making/makes* tea.
7. Ward rounds *start/are starting* at 8.
8. The nurse *smokes secretly/is secretly smoking*.
9. Sammy usually *comes/is usually coming* late.
10. One and one *makes/is making* two.
11. The doctor *checks/is checking* his patient.
12. Mary *behaves/is behaving* well today.
13. The child *always takes/is always taking* her medicine.
14. My parents *are living/live* in Amsterdam.
15. I *always burn/am always burning* my food.

1.11 Specialized Doctors

After being a junior doctor or houseman a doctor can become a senior house officer, registrar or senior registrar. Doctors can specialize in specific areas too. Then they are usually called consultants. Try to fit the different specialists into the diagram.

Puzzle

1. Doctor who specializes in paediatrics.
2. Specialist in blood disorders.
3. Expert in the interpretation of X-rays.
4. Deals with diseases that involve joints, tendons, muscles and ligaments.
5. Doctor who is specialized in the diagnosis and treatment of eye diseases.
6. Concerned with the birth of children.
7. Specialist in the structure, function and diseases of the heart.
8. Cancer expert.
9. Makes bones grow straight.
10. Specialist in diseases of women and girls, especially those affecting the female reproductive system.
11. Specializes in the study and treatment of mental disorders.
12. Works in the operating theatre.
13. Specialist in the care and treatment of old people.
14. Concerned with the diagnosis and treatment of skin disorders.

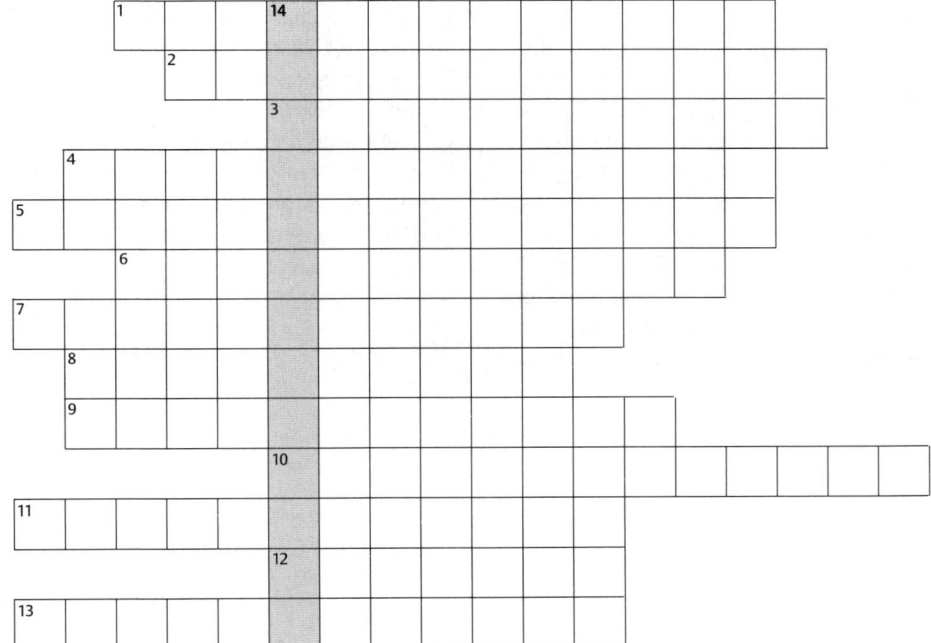

Unit 2   The Hospital

2.1 Transplant Operation

Text

Laura Davies 'critical' after second transplant

1 Five-year old Laura Davies underwent a complex 15-hour transplant operation at a hospital in Pittsburgh, in the United States, yesterday, nearly 15 months after
5 undergoing a similar operation in which she received a new liver and small intestine.

Doctors at the Children's Hospital operated to replace her stomach, large intestine,
10 small intestine, liver, pancreas and kidneys. After the operation she was said to be 'critical', on a respirator but reacting as surgeons had expected. The next 72 hours will be vital in seeing if her body will ac-
15 cept the new organs and withstand infection, Margaret Le Masters, spokeswoman for the Children's Hospital of Pittsburgh said.

Surgeons decided that the multi-trans-
20 plant was the best hope for Laura, whose body had started to reject the new organs she was given last June. Ms Le Masters said the operation went smoothly. Dr Andreas Tzakis, the surgeon, said there were
25 no complications and the procedure went more quickly than expected. Laura's small intestine transplanted last year had not been absorbing nutrition properly and was not pushing food through her body.

30 The rejection of the organ had weakened other abdominal organs.

Her surgeons felt the second transplant was her only hope of a better quality of life.
35 Laura, from Eccles, Greater Manchester, had been waiting for a suitable donor for four weeks. The hospital said the donor was of similar size and blood type.

Laura was born with a condition known
40 as short-gut syndrome that prevented her from eating normally.

Her parents, Fran and Les Davies, are waiting in the hospital during the surgery.
45 Laura's mother, Fran, aged 27, said: 'We know there are great risks involved but it's her only chance of a normal life and we have to give her that chance.'

'If we thought there was no hope she
50 would not be in there now. But if anyone can get through, Laura can.'

Laura's first transplant was funded by donations from around Britain and a contribution of more than £ 160,000 from King
55 Fahd of Saudi Arabia.

Quelle: *The Guardian* 17.11.1993

Are the following statements about the text true or false?

<table>
<tr><td></td><td></td><td>true</td><td>false</td><td>Exercise</td></tr>
<tr><td>1.</td><td>Laura is a fifteen-year-old British girl.</td><td>❏</td><td>❏</td><td></td></tr>
<tr><td>2.</td><td>It will take two days before doctors are sure that her body accepts the organs.</td><td>❏</td><td>❏</td><td></td></tr>
<tr><td>3.</td><td>Rejection and infection are the most feared complications.</td><td>❏</td><td>❏</td><td></td></tr>
<tr><td>4.</td><td>Last time Laura's body did not accept the donor organs.</td><td>❏</td><td>❏</td><td></td></tr>
<tr><td>5.</td><td>Laura had a problem with her bowels.</td><td>❏</td><td>❏</td><td></td></tr>
<tr><td>6.</td><td>The American and Saudi Arabian community contributed money for Laura's first operation.</td><td>❏</td><td>❏</td><td></td></tr>
<tr><td>7.</td><td>Laura's mother is afraid Laura is not strong enough to survive the operation.</td><td>❏</td><td>❏</td><td></td></tr>
</table>

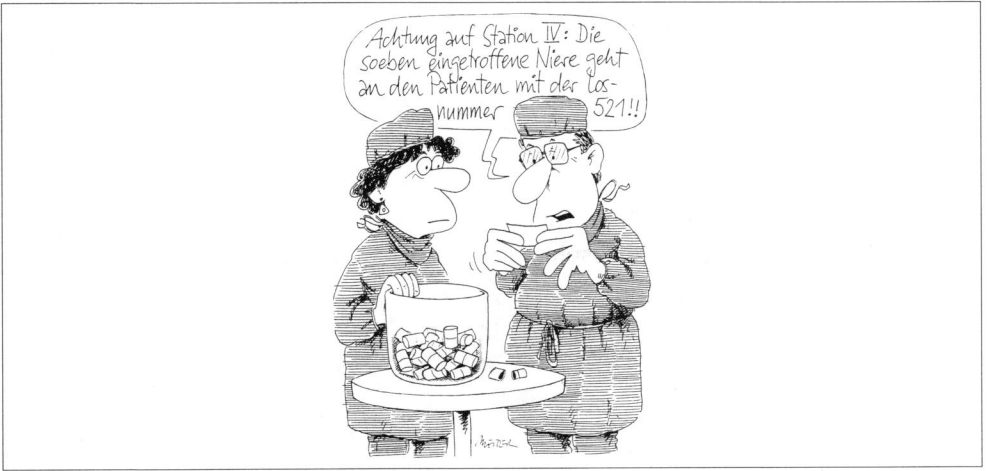

Quelle: Löwensteiner Cartoon Service (Hrsg.): Dr. med. Ironicus. Thieme, Stuttgart 1994 (S. 55)

2.2 Job Application: How to Write a Letter

Im Englischen werden Monate und Tage am Anfang stets groß geschrieben, z.B.: *Friday* 1st of *June*.

Information

Die Abkürzungen für das Datum können auf verschiedene Weise erfolgen.

Deutsch:	1. Juni 1995	oder:	01.06.1995
Englisch:	1 June 1995	oder:	1/6/1995
Amerikanisch:	June 1st 1995	oder:	6/1/1995*

* In Amerika schreibt man zuerst den Monat und dann erst den Tag, hier also aufpassen!

1. Die Anrede
   a) *wenn der Name unbekannt ist:*
      Dear Sir, Madam (UK)
      Dear Sir: Madam: (USA)
   b) *wenn der Name bekannt ist:*
      Dear Mr, Mrs, Ms, Miss, (UK)
      Dear Mr., Mrs., Ms., Miss., (USA)

2. Schlussworte:
   a) *wenn der Name unbekannt ist:*
      Yours faithfully(,) (UK)
      Yours truly (USA)
   b) *wenn der Name bekannt ist:*
      Yours sincerely(,) (UK)
      Yours truly (USA)

Sabine Mayer
Beethovenstr. 3
20251 Hamburg
Federal Republic of Germany
Tel: +49-40-3725411

1 June 1996

Personnel Department
Brookwood Hospital
Knaphill
Woking
Surrey GU2 2RQ
England

Dear Sir or Madam,

I was interested to learn from your advertisement in *Nursing Times* that ...

Yours faithfully,

[Unterschrift]

Sabine Mayer

Beispiel für die Einleitung des Briefes

Einige Beispiele:

Unter Bezugnahme auf Ihre Anzeige…	Referring to your advertisement…
Ich bewerbe mich hiermit um die Stelle als …	I wish to apply for the position of…
Ich möchte meine Kenntnisse in … erweitern	I would like to extend my knowledge of…
Meine Muttersprache ist Deutsch.	I am a native speaker of German.
Ich spreche fließend Englisch.	I speak English fluently.
In Erwartung Ihrer Entscheidung verbleibe ich…	Awaiting your decision, I remain,…

Look at the following ads in which different hospitals ask for nursing staff and see if there is a job you like. Write your application for one or more of the jobs offered.   *Exercise*

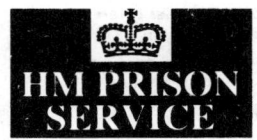

HM PRISON SERVICE

HMP BELMARSH
Western Way, Thamesmead, London SE28 0EB

Working in partnership with Oxleas NHS Trust and Thamesmead Medical Associates

GRADE E – RGN

First Level RGNs (or second level who are willing to undertake the EN conversion Course) are required to complete the multi-disciplinary Health Care Team at London's High Security Prison.

An interest in working in all fields of Prison Health Care is essential as successful candidates will rotate throughout in-patients, out-patients and residential (community) areas.

Secure unit experience would be an advantage, however, all staff are given a full supernumerary induction and training in prison work and is therefore not essential. A sense of proportion/humour is.

Salary scale £19,835 rising to £23,135 per annum (inclusive of London and Environment Allowances).

For further information/informal visits please contact Andy Barrett (Training Manager) on 020 8317 2436 extension 443 or Jan Picken (Primary Care Manager) on extension 336.

Application forms can be obtained from Karen, Recruitment and Selection, on extension 235. Fax: 020 8316 2197.

Closing date for applications – 16 March, 2001.

The Prison Service is an equal opportunities employer – we welcome applications from candidates regardless of ethnic origin, religious belief, gender, sexual orientation, disability or any other irrelevant factor.

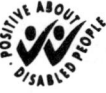

(GN6519)

Aintree Hospitals NHS Trust **NHS**
University Hospital Aintree

COMMUNITY MENTAL HEALTH SERVICES

COMMUNITY PSYCHIATRIC NURSES
E GRADE RMN

Part Time 25 hours per week, 9.30am - 2.30pm (negotiable)

How often do you feel you know exactly the job you would really love to do, the hours you would like to work and the place you would like to work in? This is it. Our roving team of CPNs is expanding. An important part of our service is the continuing care of the clients, and as part of this team, you will provide cover across the community. Your skills and experience, flexibility and adaptability will be challenged and developed with the support of continued clinical supervision and extensive training and development opportunities. We'll meet your commitment with our support.

The Trust is committed to helping staff achieve a balance between work and home life, and is implementing a range of family friendly policies. We are working together with a multi-disciplinary 'Improving Working Lives' taskforce of staff, on a range of initiatives including working practices, flexible working, valuing staff, policies and procedures.

Are you looking to return to nursing, with flexible hours? Contact Edwin Hugues-Gregoire, CPN Manager, on 0151 529 3075, for an informal discussion if you are. **Ref 519.**

F GRADE RMN
Full Time

Opportunities in our specialty teams for CPNs with a minimum of 12 months' community experience. We actively encourage and support personal professional development and offer a comprehensive package tailored to your own development plan. **Ref 517.**

Full clean driving licence essential for both posts.

Application form and job description available from Human Resources Department, Aintree House, University Hospital Aintree, Longmoor Lane, Liverpool L9 7AL. Tel. 0151 529 3905, quoting appropriate reference number.

Closing date: 15 March 2001.   (MH6585)

• *WORKING TOWARDS EQUAL OPPORTUNITIES* • *CRÈCHE* •
• *NO SMOKING POLICY IN OPERATION* • *GYM ON SITE* •

STAFF NURSES GRADES D & E

Berkshire Cancer Centre, West/Adelaide Wards

D Grade £15,000 - £16,572	Ref: D814
E Grade £16,045 - £19,370	Ref: D815

Full-time/Part-time/Night duty

An excellent opportunity has arisen for D and E Grade nurses wanting to work on a haematology/clinical oncology ward. This supportive and challenging environment would provide you with the chance to care for patients receiving high dose chemotherapy, radiotherapy, chemotherapy and symptom management. West Ward has 12 clinical oncology beds and Adelaide ward has 21 beds, incorporating 5 haematology beds in a purpose built isolation unit and 16 mixed haematology and clinical oncology beds.

For informal enquiries please contact Mary Williams on 0118 987 7454 or Lynn O'Neil on 0118 987 7471.

Please send your CV, quoting the above reference number, to Debbie Horton at the address below or telephone 0118 963 6207.

STAFF NURSE

Eye Outpatients & Casualty

Grade D/E	Ref: A831
£15,000 - £19,370 Full-time 37½ per week	

Applicants should be Eye Trained ENB 346 or have an interest in Opthalmology.

For informal enquiries please contact Jane Neal on 0118 987 7163.

Please send your CV, quoting the above reference number, to Amanda Griffiths at the address below, or telephone 0118 963 6353.

STAFF NURSE

Stubbs Ward

Grade E	Ref: C799
£16,045 - £19,370	Hours: 37½ per week

Full-time, Occasional Night Duty

You will be part of a multi-disciplinary team and need to have a minimum of one years Elderly Care experience.

Will be named nurse for 6-7 patients, so you need to be motivated, a good leader and role model.

WE OFFER • career development opportunities • free transport between hospital sites • nursery • school holiday club • subsidised staff restaurant • subsidised leisure facilities.

Working towards fairness at work

All applicants who have a disability and meet the minimum criteria for the post will be interviewed.

For informal enquiries please contact Gill Taylor on 0118 963 6329.

Please send your CV, quoting the above reference number, to Colene Waliczek at the address below or telephone 0118 963 6356.

STAFF NURSES

Head and Neck Unit

This is an exciting time to join our ENT/Aural department, soon to amalgamate with the Eye Ward to become a brand new, purpose-built Head & Neck Unit.

We are a forward thinking department, constantly reviewing and expanding nursing roles and we fully support the further training and development of our staff.

Grades D/E
ENT and Eye Wards   Ref: A818/9

£15,000 - £19,370	Full/Part-time

The department currently has vacancies for enthusiastic RGNs who would like to develop their career within this friendly, dynamic team, enjoying the benefits of clinical supervision, orientation programmes and the opportunity to rotate within department specialities.

Training opportunities offered:
• ENB 338 and ENB 998
• Encouraged to undertake extended skills, cannulation, venupuncture.

Grade F
ENT Ward   Ref: A834

£17,799 - £21,801	Full-time

Due to internal promotion we are also looking for an enthusiastic RGN for the post of Senior Staff nurse.

With at least 18 months as an E grade and ENT/maxillo facial experience, you will possess good written and verbal communication skills and the ability to work well within a multidisciplinary team. Teaching and acting as a mentor form a crucial part of this challenging role. Ideally you will possess ENB338/998 and a diploma in management or relevant supervisory experience.

Requirements and duties of the role:
• assessing, planning and evaluating patient care
• to take charge in the absence of sister
• to assist in the development of all staff.

For informal enquiries please contact Barbara McLennon on 0118 987 7488/9.

Please send your CV, quoting the above reference number, to Amanda Griffiths at the address below or telephone 0118 963 6353.

Closing date for all posts: 16th March 2001.

The Recruitment Team, Battle Hospital, Oxford Road, Reading RG30 1AG

Royal Berkshire and Battle Hospitals
NHS Trust (GN6642)

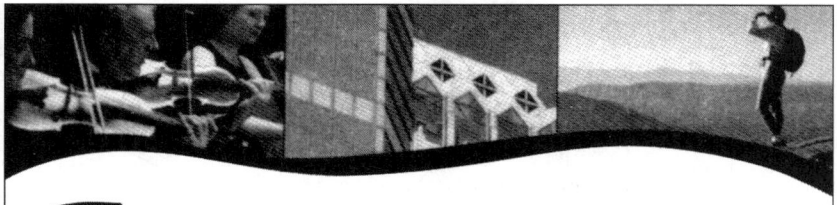

Fresno: For all the right reasons.

Say yes to Fresno, California, an "All-America City," and discover a rich array of lifestyle benefits few cities can offer! Excellent schools. Affordable neighborhoods. Abundant shopping, cultural and entertainment attractions. Fresno's central location makes it an easy choice for endless recreational adventures in neighboring mountains, beaches, national parks, major metropolitan cities and world-class destinations.

Highly competitive relocation assistance packages available.

Opportunities for British, Irish, Scottish and Canadian Nurses in California.

Move into your new career with one of California's leading healthcare centers. Immediate full-time openings for experienced nurses exist in **Coronary Care Unit, Cardiac Surgery Unit, Cardiovascular Progressive Care Unit, Cath Lab, Critical Care Unit, Post-Anesthesia Care Unit, Operating Room, Emergency Room, Medical/Oncology Unit and Surgical Unit.**

Saint Agnes Medical Center has built its reputation on providing high quality, compassionate healthcare. We are continuing our commitment to excellence by breaking ground on our largest expansion program in our 71-year history. Complete by 2003, our program will include a new state-of-the-art Heart and Vascular Center, an Imaging Department, expanded Emergency Room and Medical Education Center.

Call for a Local Interview.

If you're looking for positive change, come to Saint Agnes Medical Center. **Our recruitment consultant, Anna Stier, will be in London conducting local interviews on the following dates: Thursday, March 8 through Friday, March 9, 2001, 9:30am-6:30pm, and Saturday, March 10, 2001, 10am-5:30pm, at the Phoenix Hotel, 1-8 Kensington Gardens Square (ph: 0-207-229-2494).**

Please contact Anna Stier locally at the hotel or call 0-800-328-6648 to book an appointment. Walk-ins welcome! We are an equal opportunity employer.

Visit our website for complete details.
www.samc.com

 Saint Agnes Medical Center

(IN6475)

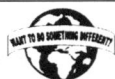
Experience spectacular desert sunsets, rugged wilderness, blue skies, lush rain forests or beautiful coastline with RALEIGH INTERNATIONAL
Nurses (aged 25+) required for three-month expeditions to:
GHANA, COSTA RICA, NAMIBIA, CHILE, BELIZE AND MONGOLIA (IN6521)

 For further information contact the Staff Office:
Tel: 020 7371 8585   Email: staff@raleigh.org.uk
Charity No 1047653

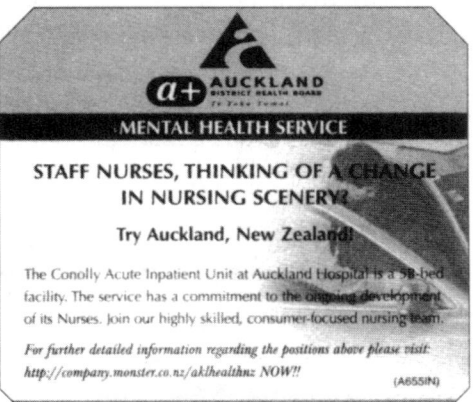

2.3 Hospital Wards

Conversation   Listen to the following conversation between a man and a nurse and then find out which ward this gentleman came from.

man: Excuse me, nurse, I was wondering whether you could help me?
nurse: Well, what seems to be the problem?
man: Actually, it's like this, I went out to buy some sweets and now I seem to be lost.
nurse: You don't remember the ward you were in?
man: That's right, but I don't think it is in this building anyway.
nurse: Why were you taken to hospital then?
man: I don't know! They said I had to because my waterworks had a small problem, but I don't think so. It's just a big fuss, that's what it is.
nurse: Can you remember when you came in?
man: No, but I know when I want to get out, that's for sure.
nurse: If you tell me your name I can go and see if the admission office knows something.
man: James, my name is James, but they usually call me Jimmy.
nurse: What about your surname, sir?
man: Well, that's Whitacker, don't you know me then?
nurse: I don't think we've met, Mr Whitacker, but if you wait here I'll see what I can do for you.
(nurse goes and returns)
nurse: It's ward 16 you're in. Come, I'll give you a hand to get there.

2.4 The Diagnosis

Information   The doctor fits together the patient's signs and symptoms to make or confirm a diagnosis. He/she starts by asking questions about current and past illnesses of the patient. This is referred to as the patient's *case history*.

When the doctor has completed the case history he/she usually continues with a physical examination. The results of the physical examination are written down under these headings:

1. inspection   2. palpation   3. percussion   4. auscultation

Choose the right definition to go with the heading.   *Exercise*

... **a)** Process of examining parts of the body by carefully feeling with the hands
   and fingertips.
... **b)** Listen to the sounds of the heart and lungs by means of a stethoscope.
... **c)** Examining by sight and observation.
... **d)** Examining parts of the body by tapping with fingers or an instrument and
   sensing the resultant vibrations.

The examination can be combined with X-rays, urine tests and blood samples.

The pictures below show basic equipment for a physical examination. What is what?   *Exercise*

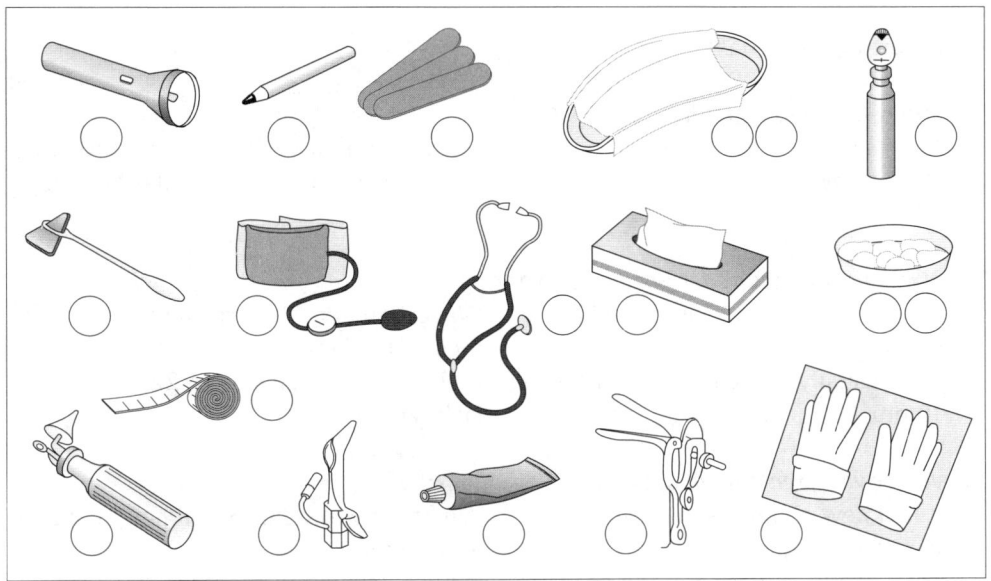

1. emesis basin/vomit bowl
2. lubricant
3. blood pressure cuff
4. glove
5. flashlight/torch
6. paper towel
7. antiseptic solution
8. percussion hammer
9. cotton balls

10. otoscope
11. skin pencil
12. stethoscope
13. ophthalmoscope
14. tissues
15. tongue depressors
16. tape measure
17. vaginal speculum
18. nasal speculum

2.5 The (Simple) Past Tense

Grammar

Das Imperfekt wird gebildet durch
- **das Verb + „*ed*"** (bei regelmäßigen Verben)
  oder
- **die Vergangenheitsform der unregelmäßigen Verben**
  (siehe Anhang A)

She worked very hard yesterday.	Sie arbeitete gestern sehr hart.
I saw him at the office last Monday.	Ich sah ihn letzten Montag im Büro.

She worked very hard yesterday.

[_____]_____._____   *Imperfekt*

         now

Diese Form gibt an, dass:

1. *etwas klar und endgültig vorbei ist*
Mary's father died last year.	Marys Vater ist voriges Jahr gestorben.
He last saw a doctor in 1990.	1990 war er zum letzten Mal bei einem Arzt.

2. *etwas normal war oder wiederholt vorkam*
We always gave the children a hot drink.	Wir gaben den Kindern stets etwas Warmes zu trinken.
They usually switched the light off at 10 pm.	Meistens machten sie um 22 Uhr das Licht aus.

3. *von etwas Irrealem die Rede ist*
If he knew about his disease, he would be desperate.	Wüsste er von seiner Krankheit, würde er verzweifeln.
They would be very angry if they knew.	Sie würden ziemlich ärgerlich werden, wenn sie davon wüssten.

Exercise

Choose the correct form.

1. Sarah *falls/fell* ill yesterday.
2. I *saw/see* him fall.
3. He *injects/injected* the wrong patient this morning.
4. I *am/was* happy when I *am/was* in Africa.
5. He always *visits/visited* his grandmother.

6. If there *was/is* more money we could ask for more staff.
7. Louis Pasteur *dies/died* in 1895.
8. The sun *rose/rises* at 6 am this morning.
9. That nurse frequently *asks/asked* for help.
10. The patient *falls/fell* off his bed.

2.6 Translation

Translate the following sentences.   *Exercise*

1. Er hat heute Nacht ausgezeichnet geschlafen.

_____

2. Die Patienten durften am Wochenende nach Hause.

_____

3. Ich hörte ein unbekanntes Geräusch in seinem Zimmer.

_____

4. Die alte Dame hat ihren Brei ganz aufgegessen.

_____

5. Er hat zum Frühstück zwei Gläser Milch getrunken.

_____

2.7 The Hospital Bed

Can you find the following objects in the picture?   *Exercise*

a) bedside table
b) over-bed table
c) signal cord (USA)/
   nurse call buzzer (UK)
d) sling
e) adhesive plaster

f) plaster (of Paris)
g) thermometer
h) rails
i) get-well card
j) bedpan

k) male urinal
l) sheet
m) charts
n) pillow
o) handgrip/trapeze

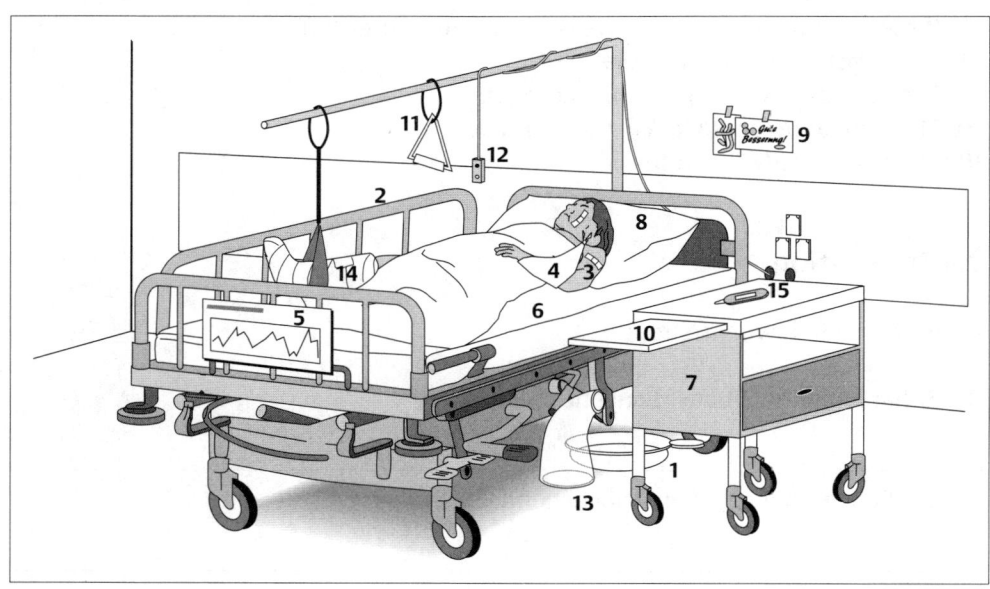

2.8 Hospital Departments

People usually go to see their GP when they have had an accident, or need advice, a check-up or medicine. Sometimes the doctor will send patients to a specialist for a second opinion or to a general hospital for tests or an operation.

A hospital is a complicated organization of units, each of which specializes in one kind of illness or treatment. Examples of departments that can be found in a general hospital are:

medical department:	cares for patients with medical conditions
surgical department:	cares for patients undergoing surgery
paediatric department:	cares for sick or injured children
obstetric department:	cares for maternity patients and the newborn
emergency department:	cares for trauma victims or victims of natural disasters or medical emergencies

There are some units in the hospital where patients only go for an examination or special treatment. Examples of these units are:

out-patients clinic:	gives specialist treatment to out-patients
renal unit:	treats patients with kidney diseases
haematology department:	examines and treats patients with blood disorders

Translate the names of the following wards. *Exercise*

1. _____ Kinderabteilung

2. _____ Wöchnerinnenabteilung

3. _____ Nierendialyse

4. _____ Erste Hilfe

5. _____ OP

6. _____ Röntgenabteilung

7. _____ Abteilung Onkologie

8. _____ Lungenabteilung

9. _____ HNO

10. _____ Abt. Chirurgie

2.9 Medical and Surgical Patients

About half of the patients in hospital usually need an operation. They are called sur- *Exercise*
gical patients and go to surgical wards. People who don't need an operation usually
go to medical wards or specialized wards. Which patient goes to which ward? (Start
with the patients.)

medical ward

... **a)** renal unit
... **b)** dermatology
... **c)** neurology
... **d)** cardiology
... **e)** haematology
... **f)** gastrointestinal
... **g)** respiratory
... **h)** general medicine
... **i)** oncology

surgical ward

... **j)** orthopaedics
... **k)** ENT (ear/nose/throat)
... **l)** general surgery
... **m)** urology
... **n)** gynaecology
... **o)** vascular surgery
... **p)** plastic surgery
... **q)** neurosurgery

Patients

1. Patient who wants a transfer of healthy tissue to repair damaged area and to restore and create form.
2. Fairly young patient suffering from sickle-cell anaemia (= inability to form normal haemoglobin).
3. Patient who needs dialysis.
4. Adult patient who needs tonsillectomy.
5. Patient who has suffered a stroke.
6. Older man who suffers from hypertrophy of the prostate gland.
7. Patient who has to be admitted for a bronchoscopy.
8. Patient with severe eczema.
9. Male patient who needs an operative treatment of his spinal cord.
10. Patient who has had a cardiac arrest.
11. Female patient who needs a D & C (= dilatation and curettage).
12. Patient who suffers from pancreatitis.
13. Young female patient with compound femur fracture.
14. Patient suffering from an autoimmune disease.
15. Patient who suffers from Hodgkin's disease.
16. Patient who needs a surgical bypass of an arterial obstruction.
17. Emergency patient for an appendicectomy (UK)/appendectomy (USA).

2.10 Word combinations

Exercise Fill in the right verb.

1. A week after the crash she _____ consciousness. (zu Bewusstsein kommen)

2. Can I _____ your blood pressure? (Blutdruck messen)

3. He _____ control when he heard the news. (die Selbstbeherrschung verlieren)

4. The doctor _____ his round. (macht Visite)

5. The district nurse _____ the baby's height. (Körpergröße messen)

6. Please _____ your breath. (Atem anhalten)

7. The man _____ a lot of pain today. (hat Schmerzen)

8. I always _____ headaches after reading. (Kopfschmerzen bekommen)

9. I _____ sick. (sich unwohl fühlen)

10. He _____ a cold in the snow yesterday. (sich eine Erkältung holen)

2.11 Assessment of Statements

Are the following statements true or false?

	true	false	Exercise
1. A *porter* is the person in charge of the entrance to a hospital.	❑	❑	
2. A doctor uses a *torch* to clog up his/her patient's ears.	❑	❑	
3. A *sphygmomanometer* [ˌsfɪgməʊməˈnɒmɪtə] in Great Britain is the same thing as a blood pressure apparatus in the USA.	❑	❑	
4. An *ambulatory* patient is a patient who is allowed and able to get up and walk around.	❑	❑	
5. PM stands for 'post meridiem', which literally means 'morning'.	❑	❑	
6. *Containment isolation* is used for out-patients.	❑	❑	
7. Deep cuts often need to be *stitched up*.	❑	❑	
8. When someone *faints* he or she needs to go to hospital immediately.	❑	❑	
9. *Vomiting* can be caused by food poisoning.	❑	❑	
10. When germs enter our blood system, lymphocytes produce chemicals called *antibodies* to fight them.	❑	❑	

Unit 3   Nursing

3.1 No Task for Nurses

Excercise

Fill in the gaps with the words on the next page.

APPENDIX NURSE QUITS

The nurse who (1) _____ an outcry after helping perform an appendix operation has quit her job. Sister Valerie Tomlinson, who received a written (2) _____ over her role in the operation, said she felt (3) _____ by some colleagues. Mrs Tomlinson, 53, was moved from the operating (4) _____ to a desk job after being allowed to return to work in January. But now she has chosen to (5) _____ early. At her home in a remote Cornish village she said: 'One of the major factors in my (6) _____ to go was the way some people treated me when I came back. I received great support from some colleagues but quite the (7) _____ from others.'

'The whole thing was a great (8) _____ ,' she said. 'What kept me going was that I had 130 (9) _____ of support from the public and only one against me. Now I just want to put the whole thing (10) _____ me.'

A disciplinary hearing was told that Mrs Tomlinson (11) _____ three elements of the operation on a man at Treliske Hospital, Truro. Under the instruction of surgeon Tahir Bhatti, she made the incision, (12) _____ the appendix and then closed the wound. She admitted her actions breached (13) _____ , and received a formal warning from the Royal Cornwall Hospitals Trust. At the same time, Mrs Tomlinson said she was looking (14) _____ to returning to her £ 18,000 job at the hospital where she had worked for 17 years. The separated mother of two said the new patients' charter had put impossible (15) _____ on nursing staff, another factor in her decision to retire.

A junior member of staff at Treliske said: 'All those I know were on her side, but perhaps some felt a bit embarrassed after what happened.' Treliske Hospital spokeswoman Jan Honey said: 'Mrs Tomlinson's decision to take early retirement was entirely her own. No pressure was put on her, and the management has given her full support.'

Quelle: *The Mail on Sunday*, 18-6-1995

1. **a)** led
   b) sparked
   c) asked for
   d) had

2. **a)** message
   b) treatment
   c) warning
   d) threat

3. **a)** let down
   b) helped
   c) warned
   d) cheered

4. **a)** ward
   b) surgeon
   c) procedure
   d) theatre

5. **a)** tired
   b) retire
   c) tyre
   d) work

6. **a)** decision
   b) pleasure
   c) cause
   d) behaviour

7. **a)** same
   b) only
   c) right
   d) reverse

8. **a)** adventure
   b) ordeal
   c) order
   d) experience

9. **a)** presents
   b) warnings
   c) letters
   d) demands

10. **a)** behind
    b) back
    c) over
    d) after

11. **a)** assisted
    b) took
    c) tore off
    d) carried out

12. **a)** cut off
    b) sawed off
    c) broke off
    d) stitched

13. **a)** the peace
    b) guidelines
    c) plans
    d) behaviour

14. **a)** back
    b) up
    c) forward
    d) for

15. **a)** questions
    b) conflicts
    c) demands
    d) outcomes

3.2 Working Shifts

Unit 1 already mentioned that nurses run hospital wards 24 hours a day. These 24 hours can be divided into *early morning care* (AM care) and *bedtime care* (PM care). The periods are usually split into 3 shifts: *early shift, back shift* and *night shift.* Nurses work according to a *roster/rota.*

Let's see what Jenny (RGN), Mike (RMN) and Jill (RNMH) did yesterday. Jenny was on an early shift, Mike worked a back shift and Jill had night duty. They speak with an interviewer (I). *Conversation*

I: Jenny, can you describe yesterday's day at work?
Jenny: I can indeed. It was one of those hectic days again, everything seemed to happen all at once. First I had to help handing out the breakfasts because both the kitchen help and the AN called in sick. While the patients were eating we went into the office and read the reports. I work at a surgical ward at the moment,

so after reading the reports I first prepared the patients who had to go in for surgery. At the same time I had to check the vital signs from patients who had been operated on the day before. I rushed around to provide wash water and toiletries for people who had to stay in bed and helped others with a bath or shower. Before I finished with all this, patients came back again from surgery. And in the afternoon we had three emergency admissions. I thought the day would never end, but fortunately we coped really well.

I: What about you, Mike, did you also have a busy day?

Mike: I work at a ward for patients with acute mental illness and although there were only ten patients, those ten kept us on our feet all right. Two of them were on close obs, which means you have to stay with them all the time so they can't harm themselves. I was assigned to look after a young man who was extremely manic. He was too agitated to go to the toilet or eat something so I had to run after him all afternoon. I tried to have a conversation with him but he just couldn't stop running up and down. In the end we had to increase his medication because he would have collapsed otherwise.

I: Was that how your night shift went as well, Jill?

Jil: Oh no, nothing like that. I work in a geriatric ward so apart from the occasional wandering patient it was fairly quiet. We had to change a few beds of patients who had wet their bed and helped others with a bedpan or urinal. But most of them were sound asleep through the night. It was very quiet really.

Exercise Translate the following words from the text.

1. _____ zuweisen

2. _____ Mittagsdienst

3. _____ glücklich

4. _____ Frühdienst

5. _____ herumgehen

6. _____ unruhig

7. _____ bettnässen

8. _____ drängen

9. _____ Bettpfanne

10. _____ erhöhen

3.3 Fluency: A patient's daily care in the general hospital

Imagine you are a qualified nurse who has to instruct a student nurse in the patient's daily care.

Exercise

The qualified nurse explains to the student nurse:

- What and how she/he has to do;
- When it should be done;
- Why it should be done;
- Where it should be done.

The tasks mentioned below should be addressed.

The student nurse asks:

- How she/he should do something;
- Anything that is not clear;
- Any other questions she/he can think of.

1. ... Wake up the patient and after checking vital signs give him/her opportunity to use the bathroom.
2. ... Check bedsores.
3. ... If permitted offer bedtime drink.
4. ... Supply breakfast and medication.
5. ... Listen to the patient's worries.
6. ... Read reports.
7. ... Provide the patient with wash water and toiletries or help the patient to the bath or shower.
8. ... Help visitors to find the right room.
9. ... Provide bedpan or urinal, assist to toilet.
10. ... Place over-bed table with a drink within reach.
11. ... Assist with mouth and hair care.
12. ... Give back rub when the patient is confined to bed and give special attention to pressure areas.
13. ... Change the patient's pyjamas or gown.
14. ... Evaluate the patient's progress.
15. ... Put bed in lowest position and side rails up.
16. ... Hand out medication if necessary.
17. ... Remove unnecessary equipment or articles from the room.
18. ... Check dressings.
19. ... Change linen if soiled.
20. ... Provide hot milk.

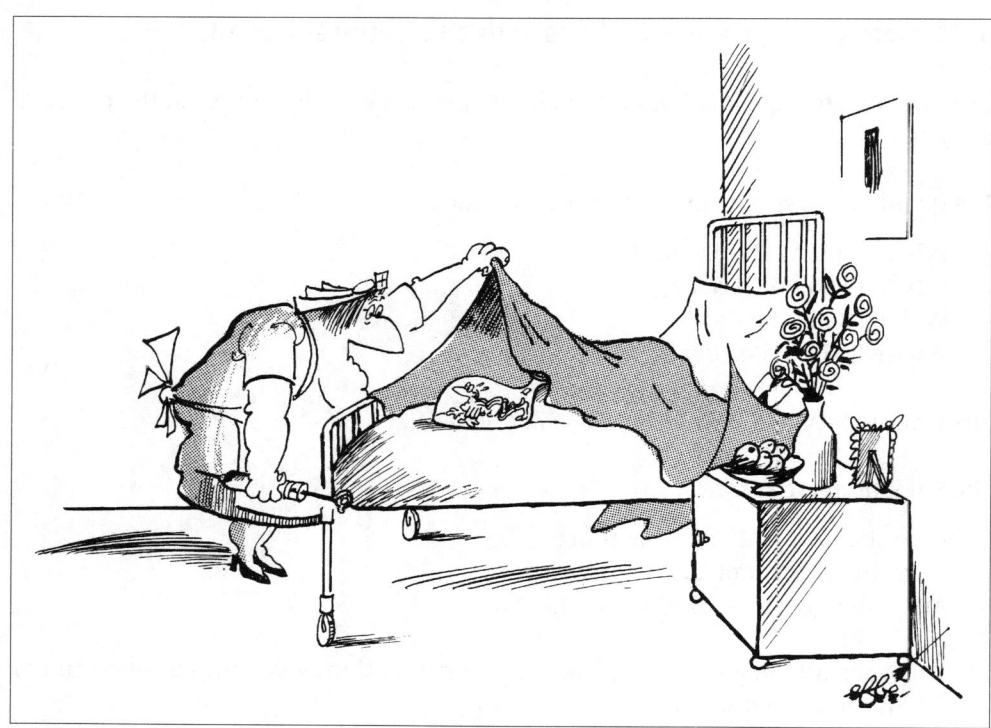

Quelle: Löwensteiner Cartoon Service (Hrsg.): Dr. med. Ironicus. Thieme, Stuttgart 1994 (S. 12)

3.4 Wound Management

Checking and changing dressings is an important daily task for nursing staff. Try to match the descriptions with the right pictures.

Exercise

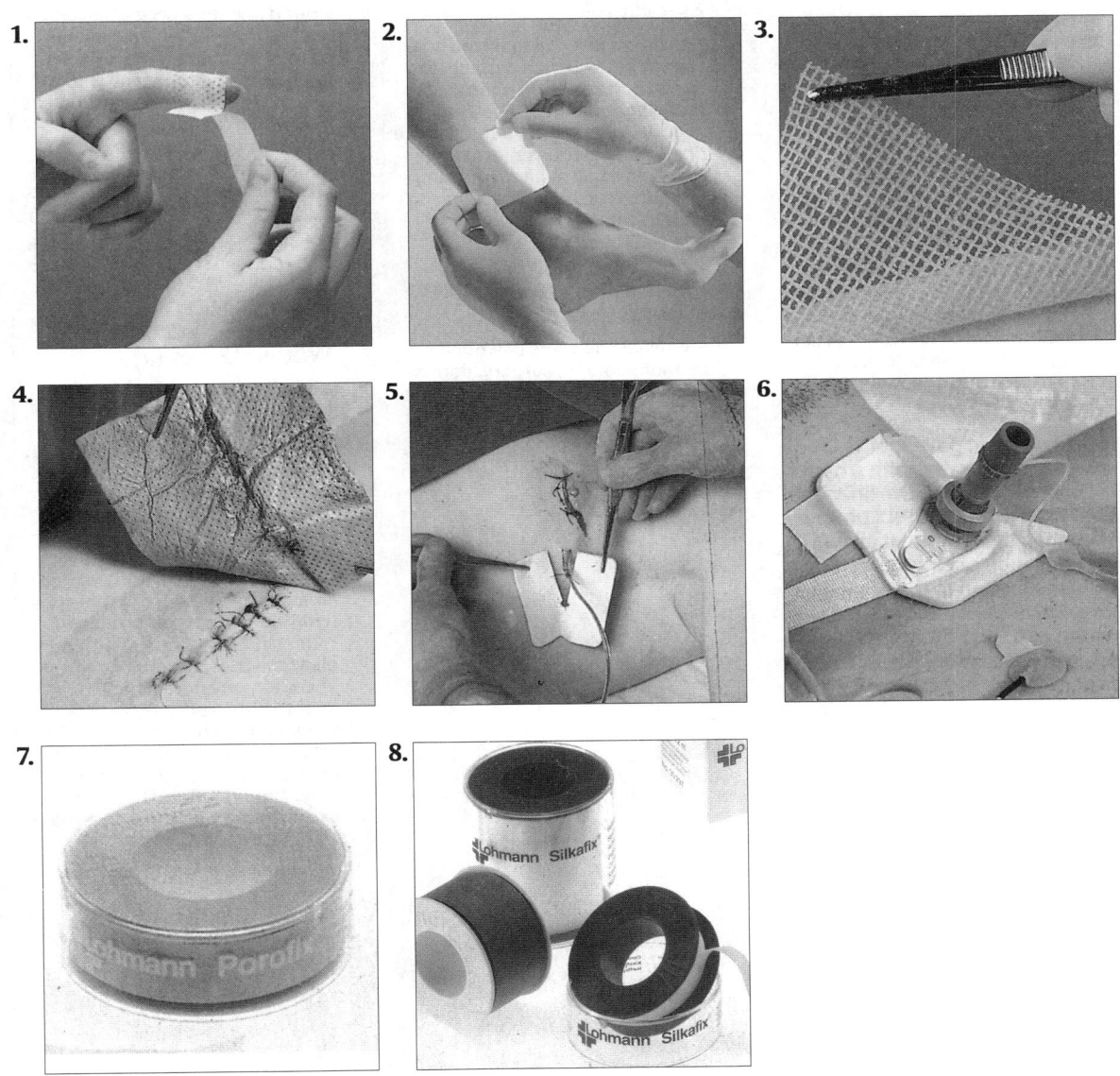

a) Metalline® Non Adherent Drainage Dressing

With pre-cut punch hole and slit, designed as a small calibre drainage dressing.

b) Curaplast® Finger Dressing

Flesh-coloured, elastic nonwoven with hypoallergenic adhesive, with Metalline® non adherent dressing pad to ensure rapid absorption of wound exudate.

c) Silkafix® Acetate Adhesive Non Stretch Tape

Coated with a hypoallergenic adhesive, water and dirt repellent. May be torn lengthwise or crosswise, indicated for use in securing: dressing pads to sensitive skin, catheters, cannulae, drainage tubes, probes.

d) Metalline® Non Adherent Tracheo Dressings

With pre-cut punch hole and slit. Designed as a tracheostomy and large calibre drainage dressing.

e) Porofix® Cotton/Rayon Adhesive Tape

Woven from cotton and spun rayon to produce a strong flesh-coloured, non stretch fabric, which is coated with zinc oxide/rubber adhesive.

f) Metalline®

Needle punched aluminized coating onto nonwoven surface. Produces non adherent, absorbent dressings with good wicking action – to keep the wound surface dry. Metalline dressings can be removed easily without sticking – important for wound healing and patient comfort.

Metalline® Non Adherent Wound Dressing

For use on all kinds of wounds in traumatology, surgery, dermatology and phlebology.
Sterile.

g) Lomatuell® H Paraffin Gauze

Loosely-woven gauze, of 100% cotton, impregnated with a hydrophobic (water-resistant) liniment base (with paraffin BP). Lomatuell H soothes the wound; it allows easy passage of exudate and good ventilation to the area, It will not stick to the surface of the wound and thus promotes rapid healing. In addition, the liniment base of Lomatuell H is in itself a sound medication for all wounds. Lomatuell H is principally used as a soothing dressing for surface wounds such as grazes, lacerations, burns, sores caused by radiation treatment and leg ulcers.
Sterile.
Individually packed to peel pouch.

h) Opragel® Hydrogel Wound Dressing

Absorbent dressing which functions on the principle of moist wound healing.
Opragel has been specially developed for the treatment of ulcera cruris, superficial decubital ulcers, superficial wounds such as skin abrasions, 1st and 2nd degree burns, skin donor sites. Opragel is a pliable, transparent laminate consisting of a film-type hydrogel wound pad produced from natural proteins, poly- and disaccharides, a synthetic water absorber, moisture maintaining agent, preservatives and 35% water. It has a plastic filmbacking that is permeable to water vapour but cannot be penetrated by bacteria. The wound pad has a protective covering which is easy to peel off before application.

Individually packed to peel pouch.

3.5 Routine Vital Signs and Weight

An important task for nurses is to monitor the patient's vital signs. These include: *Information*
- body temperature (T)
- pulse (P)
- respiration (R)
- blood pressure (BP).

The first 3 vital signs are known as *TPR values.*

Temperature

Temperature values may be expressed in either of two scales:
Fahrenheit   = F (32 ←...→ 212°) (freezing – boiling)
Celsius   = C (0 ←...→ 100°)

Normal body temperature is *98.6°F/37°C.*

Temperature is usually measured in the mouth (oral), rectum (rectal), armpit (axillary) or groin (inguinal).
Temperature variations:
axil/ing: 96.6– 98.6°F/36.1–36.9°C
oral: 97.6– 99.6°F/36.4–37.2°C
rectal: 98.6–100.6°F/36.6–37.4°C

To convert from Celsius to Fahrenheit first divide by 5 then multiply with 9 and finally add 32.
37°C → 37 : 5 → 7.4 x 9 → 66.6 + 32 → 98.6°F

To convert from Fahrenheit to Celsius subtract 32, divide by 9 and multiply with 5.
105°F → 105 – 32 → 73 : 9 → 8.11 x 5 → 40.5°C

A relatively new way of determining body temperature is by means of the *aural (ear) thermometer.* This thermometer has a built-in converter that provides the equivalent oral, rectal or axillary values in both Fahrenheit and Celsius. In addition to this thermometer there are the glass *clinical thermometers, electronic thermometers* of which the probe with disposable protective sheath is inserted into the patient and finally the *disposable oral thermometer.*

Irregularities in temperature are called:
- *fever/pyrexia* (Fieber): rise in body temperature above normal;
- *subnormal temperature* (Untertemperatur): temperature below the normal range.

Pulse

The radial measured pulse is the most commonly measured pulse. It is measured at the radial artery in the wrist. Pulse measurement includes determining the rate or speed and character (rhythm and volume) of the pulse.

Arrhythmias or irregularities in the pulse are:

bradycardia (Bradykardie): an unusually slow pulse;
tachycardia (Tachykardie): an unusually fast pulse;
sinus arrhythmia (Sinusarrhythmie): an increase of the pulse on inspiration, decrease on expiration;
extrasystole (Extrasystole): premature heartbeats due to an impulse generated somewhere in the heart outside the sinoatrial node;
pulsus bigeminus (Bigeminuspuls): double pulse wave produced by interpolation of extrasystoles (often due to excessive digitalis administration);
fibrillation (Fibrillation): totally irregular beating of the many individual muscle fibres of the heart;
heartblock (Herzblock): partial or complete impairment of conduction of the electrical impulses causing the pumping action to slow down.

Respiration

There are two parts to each respiration: one *inspiration* (inhalation), followed by one *expiration* (exhalation).
Respiration is checked for rate, rhythm, symmetry, volume and character.

Irregularities in respiration are:

tachypnoea [ˌtækɪ(p)'niːə] (Tachypnoe): rapid breathing;
dyspnoea [dɪsp'nɪə] (Dyspnoe): laboured or difficult breathing;
shallow breathing (flache Atmung): breaths that fill lungs only partially;
Cheyne-Stokes respiration (Cheyne-Stokes-Atmung): periods of dyspnoea followed by *apnoea* ['æpnɪə] or respiration stop;
stertor (Schnarchen): snoring type of noisy breathing;
rales (Röcheln): moist respirations.

Blood Pressure

BP is determined by watching the *gauge* [geɪdʒ] (meter) and listening with the *stethoscope*. The blood pressure apparatus is called a *sphygmomanometer* [ˌsfɪgməʊmə'namɪtər] or 'sphyg'.
The first regular sound is the *systolic* pressure, the last sound is the *diastolic* pressure.

Irregularities in blood pressure are:

hypertension (Hypertension): high blood pressure;
hypotension (Hypotension): low blood pressure.

Weight

Another important recording, although not one of the vital signs, is *weight*. When a patient is admitted to hospital, his or her weight is recorded. Although countries aim at one standard, British and American recordings may still differ from German weights.

German:	1 kilogram	= 2 pounds = 1000 gram
British:	1 stone	= 6.350 kilogram
	1 pound (lb)	= 0.454 gram
	1 kilo(gram)	= 2.2 pounds (lbs)
American:	1 pound (lb)	= 0.454 gram
	1 kilo(gram)	= 2.2 pounds (lbs)

3.6 Problem needs

Study the six different charts with problem needs and then try to fit in the actions that are left out.   *Exercise*

1

NAME _____   UNIT NO _____

PROBLEM/NEED

_____ Needs assistance with hygiene needs and dressing.

EXPECTED OUTCOME

_____ Will feel clean and comfortable.

ACTION	EVALU...
• Assist with a bed bath or wash as required.	
•	
•	
• Care of hair, teeth and nails as necessary.	
• Use patients own toiletries and ask carers to bring them in if possible	
• Involve carers in personal care as appropriate.	
•	
• Ensure appropriate clothes and footwear is used when the patient is out of bed.	
• Encourage the patient to help them selves whenever possible to promote independence.	

DATE _____   SIGN _____

2

NAME _____   UNIT NO _____

PROBLEM

The patient has a reduced level of mobility due to _____

EXPECTED OUTCOME

To encourage and facilitate safe mobilisation within his/her capabilities and limitations.

ACTION	EVALU...
•	
• Refer to physiotherapist and involve in the plan of care.	
• Give praise and encouragement for progress and positive achievement.	
• Assist with hygiene and toileting needs.	
• Check condition of feet and footwear.	
•	
• Use pressure relieving aids as applicable.	
•	
• Involve carers in the plan of care and keep them updated.	
• Assess home set up suitability and involve discharge teams as appropriate.	
• Administer prophylactic anticoagulation if prescribed and monitor for complications of reduced mobility.	
• Monitor for signs of constipation.	

DATE _____   SIGN _____

3

DATE _____ NAME _____ UNIT NO _____

PROBLEM/NEED

_____ Has difficulty sleeping.

EXPECTED OUTCOME

_____ Will feel safe and comfortable.

ACTION	EVALU...
• Assess normal sleep paterns	
•	
• Encourage him/her to express any fears or anxieties	
•	
• Ensure they are not too hot/cold	
• Offer drink as appropriate	
• Assess environment is conducive to sleep 1. Light 2. Mattress 3. Bed clothes 4. Position of bed on the ward 5. Noise levels	
•	
• Inform doctor of any sleep problems	
• Give support and advice as required	

4

DATE _____ NAME _____ UNIT NO _____

PROBLEM/NEED

_____ May have difficulty communicating due to illness/language barrier/disability.

EXPECTED OUTCOME

_____ Will be able to express his needs and anxieties.

ACTION	EVALU...
• Ensure call button is within reach and patient is aware how to use it	
•	
•	
• Encourage him/her to write down needs if appropriate	
• Discuss care with relatives when possible and keep them informed of patients care plan	
• Give full explanation of procedures and check understanding	
•	
• Discuss any special needs with carers	
• Obtain any special equipment from SALT or OT, check hearing aid as necessary.	

5

NAME _____ UNIT NO _____

PROBLEM/NEED

_____ Has a urinary catheter in situ.

EXPECTED OUTCOME

_____ Will feel clean and comfortable, minimise risk of infection.

ACTION	EVALU...
• Clean catheter site daily and as required.	
•	
•	
• Encourage fluids orally	
•	
• Ensure patient feels comfortable	
• Educate patient on catheter care as appropriate.	

Left out actions:

1 Maintain a safe environment at all times.
2 Offer assistance with a bath or shower and shave.
3 Give warm not hot drinks as appropriate.
4 Nurse in a comfortable position.
5 Ensure nurse call buzzer is within reach.
6 Refer to speech/language therapist.
7 Observe skin condition.
8 Give patient time to express his/her needs.
9 Empty catheter bag 4-6 hourly.
10 Maintain dignity and privacy at all times.
11 Maintain fluid balance chart.
12 Talk slowly and effectively where required.
13 Ensure patients is not in pain.
14 Monitor for signs of urine infection.
15 Ensure patient has adequate bedclothing and is in a suitable position on the ward.
16 Monitor conscious level.
17 Offer night sedation if prescribed.
18 Monitor pressure areas and encourage changes of position, whilst at increased risk.

NAME _____ UNIT NO _____

PROBLEM/NEED

_____ Has a low temperature.

EXPECTED OUTCOME

Temperature will return to within normal limits.

ACTION	EVALU...
• Nurse the patient in a comfortable position.	
•	
• Administer IV fluids (via a warmer if required)	
• Check and record temperature; half hourly, hourly, four hourly.	
•	
•	
• Monitor and record BP and pulse; half hourly, hourly, four hourly	
• Monitor and record strict fluid balance.	
• Assess waterlow score and take appropriate action if at risk.	
• Aim to disturb or expose patient as little as possible.	
• Monitor conscious level.	
• Give reassurance and maintain the patients dignity at all times.	

DATE _____ SIGN _____

3.7 Dressing and Undressing the Patient

Text

Directions for helping a patient dress after a bath

1 If possible allow the patient to select clothing. Cover patient with bath blanket and place top bedclothes on foot of bed. Bra: slip straps over patient's hands and
5 move straps up arms and position on shoulders, hook bra. Undershirt/vest or any garment that slips over the head: slip over patient's head, grasp patient's hand and guide it through
10 arm hole. Assist patient to sit forward, adjusting vest so it is smooth and over upper body. Underwear/slacks/underpants/briefs/panies: slip underwear over feet and draw
15 up the legs as high as possible. Assist patient to raise buttocks and draw garment over buttocks and up around waist. Fasten garment if necessary. Shirt/blouse, cardigan: insert your hand
20 through sleeve and grasp hand of patient, drawing sleeve over your hand and patient's. Adjust sleeve at shoulder and assist patient to sit forward so you can arrange clothing across back. Repeat this
25 on the other side. Button, zip or snap garment. Pantyhose/tights: gather pantyhose and adjust over toes and feet. Draw up over feet and legs as high as possible. Assist
30 patient to raise hips and position pantyhose. Socks: roll socks and adjust over toes, draw up over foot. Adjust so socks lie flat and smooth.
35 Shoes/slippers: slip shoe on, use shoehorn if necessary.

40 Quelle: Hegner and Caldwell, *Nursing Assistant*

Translate the following words from the text.

Exercise

1. _____ Ärmel

2. _____ Weste

3. _____ BH

4. _____ Hemd

5. _____ Pantoffeln

6. _____ hochziehen/aufrichten

7. _____ Schuhlöffel

8. _____ Hose

9. _____ (fest) ziehen

10. _____ Kleidungsstück

3.8 The Present Perfect Tense

Das englische Perfekt hat im Deutschen zwei mögliche Übersetzungen:
Perfekt oder „seit" + Präsens

Diese Zeitform wird im Englischen gebildet durch:
„have/has" + Partizip (siehe Anhang A).

Peter has broken his leg.	Peter hat sein Bein gebrochen.
I have worked as a midwife since 1990.	Ich arbeite schon seit 1990 als Hebamme.

____[1990_____.]_____ Perfect
                    now

Diese Form gibt an, dass:

1. *auf eine nicht näher definierte Vergangenheit verwiesen wird*

Have you ever nursed hemiplegic patients?	Haben Sie jemals Patienten mit halbseitiger Lähmung gepflegt?
I've worked there only once.	Ich habe dort nur einmal gearbeitet.

2. *etwas in der Vergangenheit geschehen ist und nun Wirkung zeigt*

The girl has recovered from her illness.	Das Mädchen ist von seiner Krankheit genesen.
The patients have gone to bed.	Die Patienten sind zu Bett gegangen.

3. *etwas in der Vergangenheit begonnen hat und nun noch andauert, unter Angabe der Zeitdauer*

I haven't seen a doctor since last week.	Ich habe seit der vorigen Woche keinen Arzt mehr gesehen.
Sister has worked in this ward for 15 years.	Die Oberschwester arbeitet schon seit 15 Jahren in dieser Abteilung.

Choose the correct form.

[_____] _____.____ past   ___ [_____._] _____ perfect
        now   *now*

1. I *have lived/lived* here for one year now.
2. How long *were you/have you been* tube-fed when you were in hospital?
3. I *lent/have lent* her a uniform last month.
4. Her father *has been/was* dead for years.

5. I *have checked/checked* her BP every 4 hrs up until lunch.
6. Her baby *was born/has been born* too early.
7. The patient *has just come in/just came in*.
8. Who *called/has called* a minute ago?
9. *Did you see/Have you seen* your charge nurse this morning?
10. All the student nurses *were transferred/have been transferred* to Victoria Hospital.

3.9 Translation

Translate the following sentences.   *Exercise*

1. Dieses Krankenhaus wurde im vorigen Jahrhundert gebaut.

_____

2. Wir haben sie schon gekannt, als sie noch ein kleines Mädchen war.

_____

3. Ich habe ihn jede Stunde kontrolliert.

_____

4. Ich habe gestern einen Kolben mit Blut fallen lassen.

_____

5. Haben Sie die schlechte Nachricht schon gehört?

_____

3.10 Twelve Activities of (Daily) Living (A[D]LS)

Roper (1976) listed the following twelve activities of daily living.   *Exercise*

... **a)** maintaining a safe environment   ... **g)** personal cleansing and dressing
... **b)** communication   ... **h)** breathing
... **c)** expressing sexuality   ... **i)** elimination
... **d)** working and playing   ... **j)** mobilization
... **e)** resting and sleeping   ... **k)** controlling body temperature
... **f)** eating and drinking   ... **l)** dying

Which set of problems effects the ADLS mentioned above? Try to find the right combination.

1. insomnia, restlessness, pain or discomfort, anxiety, disturbances
2. SOB (shortness of breath), oxygen by nasal cannula and excessive mucus secretion
3. expression of sexual fears or anxiety, lack of privacy, sexual advances
4. physically active, overactivity, inactivity, bedsores, thrombophlebitis, contractures, lack of physiotherapy
5. difficulties in interpersonal and social relationships
6. lack of information, confusion, poor eyesight or hearing, administration of wrong medication
7. choking, diarrhoea, malnutrition, excessive alcohol consumption
8. slurred speech, illiteracy, language barrier
9. constipation, incontinence, use of catheter, need for retraining of bladder, lack of fluid control
10. terminal illness, 5 stages of grief: denial, anger, bargaining, depression, acceptance, last rites
11. loss of self-help skills, embarrassment, confusion, weakness, contractures
12. flushing, excessive perspiration, gooseflesh, shivering, hypothermia

3.11 Questions and Answers

Grammar

Um einen Satz in Fragestellungen zu bringen, haben einige englische Hauptverben das Hilfsverb „*to do*" nötig.

Sie arbeitet dort.	She works there.
Arbeitet sie dort?	*Does* she work there?

Wenn die Verben „*to be*", „*to have*" und eine Anzahl anderer Verben wie „*can, should, could*" im Satz vorkommen, so ist dies nicht nötig.

Sie ist Ärztin.	She is a doctor.
Ist sie Ärztin?	*Is* she a doctor?
Sie können mir helfen.	You can help me.
Können Sie mir helfen?	*Can* you help me?

In der Antwort wird das gleiche Verb aufgegriffen.

Does she work there? Yes, she *does*.
Is she a doctor? Yes, she *is*.
Can you help me? Yes, I *can*.

Bei einer verneinenden Antwort wird „*not*" hinter das Verb gesetzt. (Dieses wird häufig mit „*n't*" abgekürzt.)

No, she *does not/doesn't*.
No, she *is not/isn't*.
No, I *cannot/can't*.

Change the following statements into a question and respond with the already indi- *Exercise*
cated correct answer. First look at the example.

A Foley catheter contains a balloon surrounding the neck. (yes)
Does a Foley catheter contain a balloon surrounding the neck?
Yes, it does.

1. A heel protector is used to prevent pressure sores on the arms. (no)

_____

2. Synthetic sheepskin should be placed on/in places where excess pressure may be expected. (yes)

_____

3. An egg-crate mattress adds comfort. (yes)

_____

4. A bedcradle prevents the weight of the bed-side table. (no)

_____

5. Sims' position is a left lateral position often used for enema administration. (yes)

_____

6. Liquid food contains a lot of fibre. (no)

_____

7. Nauseous patients should be nursed in a horizontal position. (no)

_____

8. Patients are usually placed on NPO (nothing/nil by mouth) before an operation. (yes)

_____

9. Patients with a fractured jaw are often fed with a feeding cup or straw. (yes)

_____

10. A walker provides support to the patient's stability. (yes)

_____

3.12 Nursing

Puzzle Try to fit the English translations of the following words into the diagram.

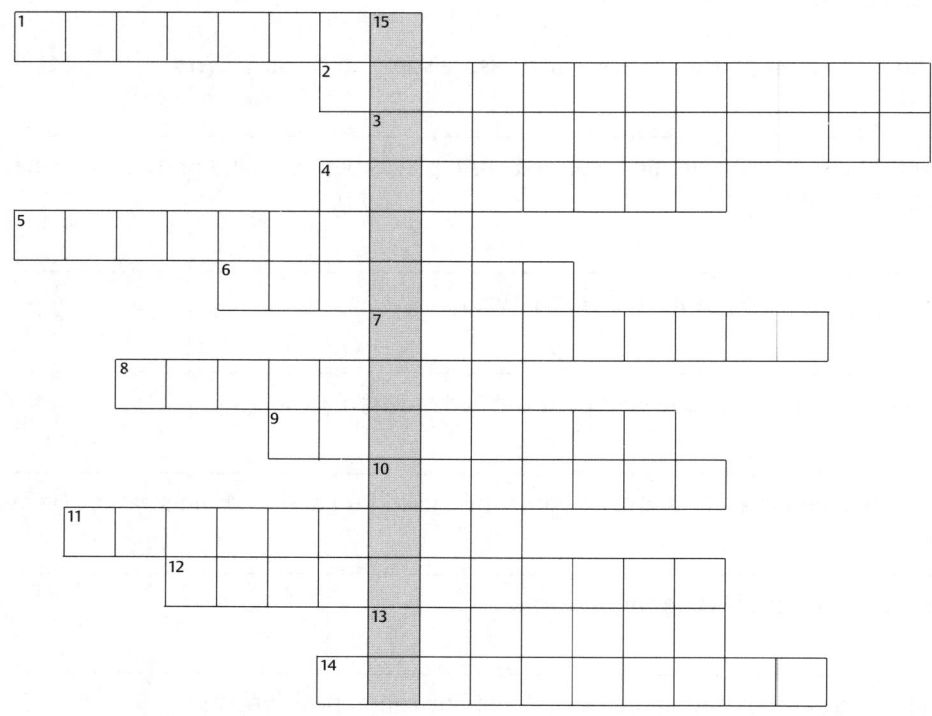

1. Schlaflosigkeit
2. Inkontinenz
3. Teamleiter
4. kg
5. Deckenbogen
6. Besteck
7. Aufnahme
8. wundgelegene Stellen
9. Chemische Reinigung
10. Nachthemd
11. Arbeitsweise
12. Wahrnehmung
13. Atem anhalten durch Schnarchen
14. Schnabeltasse
15. Pflegehilfe

Illness

4.1 Illness in Life

Text

1 **Stop behaving like hypochondriacs**

Americans poll themselves too much, and it probably creates more anxiety than en-lightenment. As the conservative writer
5 Peggy Noonan puts it: 'People who take their pulse too often are likely to make it race; people obsessed with breathing are likely to stop. Nations that use polls as daily temperature readings inevitably get
10 inauthentic readings and wind up not reassured but demoralized.'
The presumption that life can or should be pain-free is a juvenile belief. Life is in-evitably pain-inducing, and that brings us
15 back to the disease-immune system simile. The common cold afflicts millions of Americans, and most recover from it just fine. Something similar might be argued about a lot of America's maladies.
20 As the 13-year-old in my life reminds me when most problems arise, the wisest response is often very simple: 'Chill, dad.'

Quelle: 'Chill, dads – and Moms too',
us News & World Report

Match the words from the text with their translations.

Exercise

1. behaving (l. 1)	… **a)** wahrscheinlich
2. anxiety (l. 3)	… **b)** unvermeidlich
3. likely (l. 6)	… **c)** Annahme
4. inevitably (l. 9)	… **d)** kindlich
5. presumption (l. 12)	… **e)** ermunternd
6. juvenile (l. 13)	… **f)** getragen
7. inducing (l. 14)	… **g)** betasten
8. afflicts (l. 16)	… **h)** leiden
9. maladies (l. 19)	… **i)** abkühlen
10. chill (l. 22)	… **j)** Besorgnis

4.2 Waiting Room

Conversation

Mrs Dobs: Oh, hello Sarah, what brings you here? Anything wrong, dear?

Sarah: Good morning, Mrs Dobs. It's the same old problem again. I'm fine during the winter, but in spring it starts and only gets worse in summer. I just can't carry enough hankies, I'm sneezing all day.

Mrs Dobs: I know what you mean, dear. My Jerry used to be like that. He always got very grumpy at that time of year. Look who is there, it's old Tom coming this way. What's he up to this time? I bet he's been hitting the bottle again. Good morning Tom, how are you today?

Tom: What's it to you, you nosy woman! You are always poking into other people's business. You must come here every day so you don't miss any gossip, eh?

Mrs Dobs: How rude of you! I do no such thing.

Tom: Well, let's have it then. What's wrong with you this time? Yeah, that's right, you can tell us about your own little problems before we tell you anything. And why are you all flushed?

Mrs Dobs: It's a rather delicate subject which I do not wish to discuss.

Tom: Sitting on a bunch of piles again, are we? It's your own fault, sitting in your chair all day eating chocolates.

Mrs Dobs: No, I'm not. It's quite a natural problem I'm dealing with, but you men are simply not able to understand these things.

Tom: Come on Sarah, what do you think? You're a woman as well, you should know about these things.

Sarah: I don't know, Mr O'Grady, but I don't think she wants to talk about it.

Tom: Oh, rubbish, I want to know it now. Give us a hint.

Mrs Dobs: I will only say it's very normal for a woman of my age. The doctor is just giving me some medication to help me cope with it. What about you then? Why are you here?

Tom: Yeah, you would want to know that, won't you? Well, I will be as secretive as you are. I came here because the doctor said he's giving me some pills to keep me off the booze. Some wonderpills that will be!

Mrs Dobs: Well, that's very good of him. I think it's my turn now. Goodbye Sarah, bye Mr O'Grady.

Exercise

Choose the correct answer to the following questions about the conversation.

1. What does Sarah suffer from? *a cold / hay fever / flu*
2. A hankie refers to: *handkerchief / tissue / hankering*
3. What is Mrs Dobs's problem? *diabetes / menopause / overweight*
4. Piles are: *haemorrhoids / haemorrhages / hemispheres*
5. Mr O'Grady is probably getting *Vitamin B / Antabuse / antacids*

4.3 Illness in General

Information

Causes: Illnesses are caused or influenced by many factors. The causes or etiology of the illness can be *exogenous* (outside the person's body) or *endogenous* (within the person's body).

Factors that contribute to the development of a disease or illness are:
- traumas (car accident)
- pathogenic micro-organisms (bacteria)
- radiation (radioactive substances)
- allergies (asthma)
- tumors (cancer)
- psychological factors (depression)
- malnutrition (beriberi)
- chemical reactions (toxic substances)
- metabolic disorders (diabetes)
- congenital abnormalities (Huntington's disease).

Signs and *symptoms:* A *symptom* is an indication of a disease or disorder noticed by the patient. It is a subjective complaint. Examples are:
- pain
- nausea
- dizziness
- anxiety.

A *sign* is an indication of a particular disorder that is usually observed by medical staff but is not necessarily apparent to a patient. It is an objective observation. Examples are changes in:
- skin colour
- pulse, blood pressure, temperature, respiration
- character or amount of fluid intake/output
- speech, responsiveness or movement
- bodily discharge
- behaviour.

Course: The course of a disease can vary greatly. There are *acute* and *chronic* diseases.
An *acute disease:*
- starts with acute conditions
- progresses rapidly
- lasts a predictable period
- ends with recovery.

A *chronic disease:*
- has chronic conditions
- covers a prolonged period
- has periods with few signs and symptoms
- has consequences which are serious in the long term.

Exercise   Fill in one of the following words:

remission   complication   exacerbation   convalescence   relapse

Sometimes disease symptoms return after an apparent recovery has been achieved. This is called a (1) _____. Examples of illnesses that are known for their relapse are tuberculosis, gallstones/biliary colics, typhoid fever. In some cases the disease is characterized by a quiet period or (2) _____. Remission refers to a lessening in the severity of symptoms or temporary disappearance. The remission period is often interrupted by an (3) _____, a period in which the symptoms are increased. A (4) _____ is a disease or condition that arises during the course of or as a consequence of another disease. Examples of diseases that are notorious for their complications are: inflammation of the ear/otitis media → deafness, thrombosis → embolism, angina pectoris → cardiac arrest. (5) _____ is the period after an illness before achievement of the previous health status.

4.4 Different Illnesses

Exercise   Fill in the gaps with the words below.

Most illnesses take some time to secure their hold on the body. This is called the (1) _____. The human body is prepared for an invasion of (2) _____ and starts to (3) _____ them immediately. This is done by a network of organs and chemicals called (4) _____, which destroys and controls germs. (5) _____ is a very common symptom of various illnesses. It means that all the solid waste inside the bowel has become runny and liquid. A

(6) _____ is caused by pressure around the brain. An example of a visible symptom is a (7) _____. This is a skin irritation caused by an infection or allergy. A very serious disease is (8) _____, which refers to the uncontrolled division and spread of faulty cells in the body, which destroys healthy cells. (9) _____ is another serious disease. It attacks the immune system, leaving the sufferer unable to fight the (10) _____. It is easily (11) _____ sexually or by drug addicts sharing needles. (12) _____ is an example of a (13) _____. The sufferer has a congenital blood coagulation defect. A (14) _____ is a disease resulting from dietary deficiency of any substance essential for good health. (15) _____ are illnesses that spread from one person to another. Examples are (16) _____, _____, _____. Occupational disease or (17) _____ affects workers in mines, chemical plants, factories and anywhere where there is a risk of breathing in excessive amounts of (18) _____ or (19) _____ over a number of years. A well-known example of this is (20) _____, also known as silicosis and common among miners.

headache   infection   dust   deficiency disease   the immune system   AIDS flu/mumps/measles   pneumoconiosis   germs   diarrhea   chemical pollution the incubation period   haemophilia   fight   rash   cancer   transmitted   industrial disease   infections   hereditary disease

4.5 The (Present) Future Tense

Die Zukunft wird durch **„shall/will"** + **Vollverb** gebildet.

The operation will start at eight.	Die Operation wird um 8.00 Uhr beginnen.
We shall see what happens.	Wir werden sehen, was geschieht.

the operation will start at eight

_____._____[_____]__ *Zukunft*

       now

Diese Form gibt an, dass:

etwas zu einem bestimmten oder unbestimmen Zeitpunkt in der Zukunft erfolgt

He will be put on antibiotics tomorrow.	Er beginnt morgen mit einer Antibiotikakur.
From now on we shall be more careful.	Ab jetzt werden wir vorsichtiger sein.

Besonderheiten:

„Shall" wird in der Zukunft lediglich in der ersten Person Singular *(I)* und Plural *(we)* verwendet. Neben der Zukunft kann „shall" auch eine Willensäußerung wiedergeben. Dies bleibt jedoch nicht auf die erste Person beschränkt,

It shall be done.	Es wird durchgeführt werden (Ich versichere Ihnen dies).

„Will" kann für alle Personen verwendet werden. „Will" kann neben der Zukunft auch eine Willensäußerung und die Wahrscheinlichkeit für eine Tatsache ausdrücken.

Boys will be boys.	Jungen bleiben Jungen.

Sowohl „shall" als auch „will" wird mit „'ll" abgekürzt:

I'll = I will/I shall	...

Die Vergangenheit von „shall" lautet „should", die von „will" lautet „would".
Diese Formen haben eine besondere Bedeutung: „should" = Verpflichtung
„Would" verweist normalerweise in die Vergangeheit.

You should not say that.	Das solltest du nicht sagen.
When we were children we would be in and out the hospital.	Als Kinder waren wir oft im Krankenhaus.

Fill in the right tense.

1. I _____ you in five minutes. (helfen)

2. New medication _____ at 6 pm. (ankommen)

3. This patient _____ our ward soon. (verlassen)

4. I _____ to do my best. (versuchen)

5. The doctor _____ here in half an hour. (sein)

6. When _____ you _____ to our hospital? (kommen)

7. _____ we _____ now? (gehen)

8. When _____ she _____ from her operation? (zurückkommen)

9. You _____ not _____ so many questions. (fragen)

10. They _____ _____ him if they could. (helfen)

4.6 Translation

Translate the following sentences.

1. Die Patientin sagt, dass sie es tun wird.

_____

2. Wir werden Sie anrufen.

_____

3. Der Chirurg wird ihn morgen operieren.

_____

4. Die Impfung wird für Immunität gegen die Krankheit sorgen.

_____

5. Er wird schnell Ausschlag bekommen.

_____

4.7 Infections

Cause: Infections are caused by four main kinds of *germs.* These are viruses, bacteria, protozoa and fungi. Not only germs, but also worms may cause infections.

- A *virus* is a minute particle that is capable of replication but only within living cells. Viruses are too small to be visible with a light microscope. Different viruses cause illnesses including herpes, influenza, polio, AIDS and rabies.
- A *bacterium* is a single-celled creature found everywhere. They reproduce by simple division of cells. Some parasitic bacteria cause disease by producing poisons (endotoxin). An example is Salmonella bacteria.
- A *fungus* is a low form of vegetable life including yeasts, mould and mushrooms. A common fungal infection is ringworm, also known as tinea.
- *Protozoa* are single-celled animals. Most of them are harmless but some species can cause serious diseases like malaria or dysentery.
- *Worm* infections occur especially in overcrowded, unhygienic places. The roundworm, for example, affects one out of every four persons worldwide.

Infections can be spread by:
- droplet method (when viruses are in drops of liquid in a person's breath): whooping cough
- direct contact: herpes simplex
- sexual intercourse: AIDS
- water/food: cholera
- vector method (by insects): the plague.

4.8 Tropical Diseases

The two main problems in less well-developed countries are nutritional deficiency and infectious diseases. These two strongly interact. The most common *nutritional-deficiency diseases* are:
- *kwashiorkor:* features: anaemia, oedema, loss of appetite, diarrhoea, general discomfort and apathy, especially in children between 1-3 years
- *marasmus:* features: body weight below 75% of that expected for age, infant looks old, pallid, apathetic, lacks skin fat and has subnormal temperature
- *xerophthalmia/vitamin A deficiency:* features: dry, thickened and wrinkled cornea and conjunctiva
- *rickets/vitamin D deficiency:* features: misshapen bones and enlargement of wrist and ankle bones
- *scurvy/vitamin C deficiency:* features: fatigue, haemorrhage, swollen bleeding gums, rash of tiny bleeding spots on the skin around hair follicles

- *beriberi/vitamin B (thiamine/B1) deficiency:* features: pain from neuritis, paralysis, muscular wasting, progressive oedema, mental deterioration and finally heart failure
- *pellagra/vitamin B (niacin) deficiency:* features: glossitis, dermatitis, diarrhoea, weakness, mental confusion, anaemia
- *anaemia:* features: pallor, shortness of breath, tiredness, rapid pulse, swollen feet.

Other common tropical diseases are:
- malaria
- sickle-cell disease (inheritance)
- cardiac and respiratory diseases (asthma)
- tuberculosis
- disturbed consciousness, fits and epilepsy
- eye diseases (conjunctivitis)
- skin conditions (impetigo [ˌɪmpəˈtɪːgəʊ], boils, abscesses)
- leprosy
- diarrhoea
- dehydration
- worms/helminths (whipworm)
- schistosomiasis (parasitic worm infection)
- liver diseases (hepatitis)
- sexually transmitted diseases (syphilis).

4.9 Disease and Description

Try to find the right word for these definitions or descriptions of various diseases. *Exercise* Start with the definitions.

1. An acute infectious disease, primarily affecting children, due to infection of the mucous membranes lining the air passages by the bacterium *Bordetella pertussis.*
2. Sexually transmitted disease (STD) causing a burning feeling when urinating because of inflammation of the urethra.
3. Extreme and preventable deficiency disease caused by inadequate nourishment of any kind.
4. Infectious virus disease affecting the central nervous system. Immunization using Sabin vaccine is highly effective.
5. A common yeast infection of moist areas of the body, usually caused by *Candida albicans.* It is common in the mouth, skin folds and vagina, where it is known as thrush.
6. A disorder of carbohydrate metabolism in which sugars in the body are not oxidized to produce energy, due to lack of the pancreatic hormone insulin.

7. A malignant disease of the bone marrow, arising from plasma cells.
8. Swelling in the neck due to enlargement of the thyroid gland which may be due to lack of dietary iodine.
9. A yellowing of the skin or whites of the eyes, indicating excess bilirubin in the blood.
10. Term commonly used for the seizures of epilepsy.

... **a)** whooping cough/pertussis
... **b)** poliomyelitis
... **c)** fit
... **d)** diabetes mellitus
... **e)** gonorrhoea/clap
... **f)** jaundice
... **g)** malnutrition
... **h)** candidosis
... **i)** multiple myeloma
... **j)** goitre/struma

4.10 Proverbs

Exercise

A proverb is a short traditional saying, expressing a truth or moral instruction. A lot of proverbs both in English and German refer to illnesses or parts of the body but they cannot always be translated literally. Here are some examples.
Try to find the right translation for the following proverbs.

1. To be frightened to death.
2. To hate someone's guts.
3. He was beaten black and blue.
4. To be at a loss what to do.
5. With all one's heart.
6. To go off one's head.
7. To be in stitches.
8. Give someone the kiss of life.
9. To be flabbergasted.
10. To have great doubts about something.

... **a)** Sich kranklachen.

... **b)** Große Bedenken haben.

... **c)** Verrückt werden.

... **d)** Nicht mehr weiterwissen.

... **e)** Zu Tode erschrocken sein.

... **f)** Jemanden auf den Tod nicht ausstehen können.

... **g)** Verblüfft sein.

... **h)** Von ganzem Herzen.

... **i)** Er war grün und blau geschlagen.

... **j)** Jemandem Mund-zu-Mund-Beatmung geben.

5.1 AIDS Prevention

Text

Coming good with slogans

1 It's not easy getting people to change their habits, as health education experts happily tell you. Nevertheless, the 'Don't die of ignorance' campaign, mounted to counteract the spread of AIDS in this country, can claim some success.

All those adverts depicting tombstones and dead bodies may have been controversial,
5 graphic and frightening but, as Dr Eileen Rubery, head of the Department of Health's health promotion division, told last week's Annual AIDS Workshop in Brighton, the disease, although still spreading in a worrying way among heterosexuals, is now far less of a problem in
10 Britain compared to other European countries. This was not the case a few years ago.

And I like to think that wit played some role in this encouraging trend. Take the poster of a syringe beside an arm that warns: 'It only takes one prick to give you AIDS.'
15 Gets to the point, doesn't it?

However, the best poster of all – at least according to Dr Rubery, whose husband thought of it and who thinks it's 'rather brilliant' – is destined never to be seen by the British public. The slogan is simple: 'Come with a con-
20 dom'.

'The trouble is, I've never been able to get the idea past Ministers,' said a mournful Dr Rubery. Can't think why.

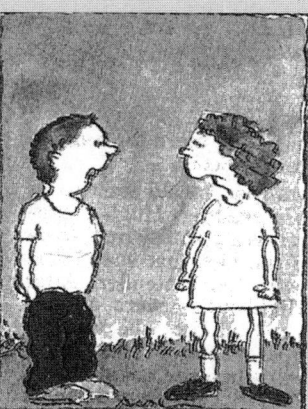

Now I know all about the birds, the bees and the viruses!

Quelle: *The Observer*, 19-9-1993

Exercise

What is the right meaning? Choose the correct answer.

1. A *habit* is: a tendency to behave in a particular way/a ritual.
2. *Nevertheless* means: not ever/in spite of that.
3. *Ignorance* means: to take no notice/lack of knowledge.
4. *Counteract* means: to reduce the effect by opposite action/to move in order to defend.
5. *Wit* means: something clever and amusing/sensibility.
6. A *syringe* is a: needle/hollow tube in which liquid can be sucked.
7. *Encouraging* means: causing feelings of courage, hope and confidence/showing courage.
8. *Mournful* means: angry/sad.

5.2 Preventative Medicine

Researchers and medical staff spend much of their time looking for ways of controlling and wiping out illness. This is just as important as curing disease, because the proverb still goes: *prevention is better than cure.*

Information

Important aspects of preventative medicine are: providing clean drinking water, introducing effective disposal of sewage, regular medical check-ups and immunization. The *World Health Organization* (WHO) deals with the state of health of people all over the world. It gives specialist advice, campaigns to control infections and organizes educational programmes.

On a regional level *health officers* from different countries are appointed by their governments to check conditions on health, hygiene and safety and implement immunization schemes. All babies are born with some immunity to disease which is passed on from their mother through the placenta. After this immunity wears off, the baby, when it is about six months old, can only become immune by suffering a disease or through vaccination.

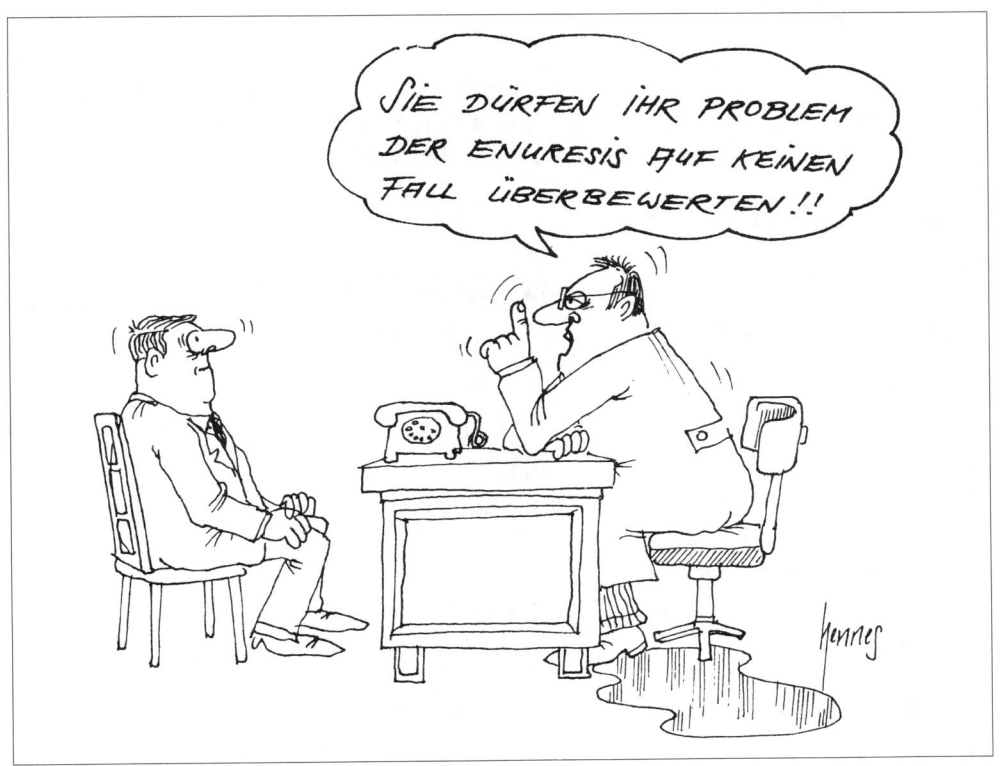

Quelle: Löwensteiner Cartoon Service (Hrsg.): Dr. med. Ironicus. Thieme, Stuttgart 1994 (S. 33)

Use these words to fill the gaps:

inherited immunity immunization immune acquired developed born susceptible

An (1) _____ person is someone who is not (2) _____ to a particular disease. (3) _____ is the state of insusceptibility to disease; we are

(4) _____ with some degree of immunity to many diseases. Natural immunity refers to (5) _____ immunity, with which a person is born. Acquired

immunity is (6) _____ in different ways during life. (7) _____ is

the process by which immunity is (8) _____ or conferred.

5.3 Immunization

Information   One of the most important parts of preventative medicine is immunization against disease. The vaccine that is given produces antibodies to kill particular germs. Vaccinations might be given by an injection, a puncher, tablets, or drops on sugar lumps.

Immunization schedule

Vaccine	Method	Age	Dose no.
DTP vaccine (diphtheria, pertussis, tetanus)	SC/IM injection	2 months	1
		3 months	2
+	oral	4 months	3
Polio	injection		
Hib vaccine (Haemophilus influenzae)			
MenC (Meningococcal C)			
MMR vaccine (measles, mumps, rubella)	IM injection	12–15 months	1
booster (diphtheria, tetanus, polio)	SC/IM injection	3 years > primary course 3 years > primary course	2
BCG	percut.id/ ID r. shoulder	babies at risk/ 10–14 years	

Vaccine	Method	Age	Dose no.
Hepatitis B	IM injection	at birth if at high risk, 1 mnth + 2 mnth, booster at 12 mnths	1

Note: Not all countries have the same schedule.
Source: Nursing Times February 17 – 2000, Vol. 96, nr. 7

5.4 Modal Auxiliaries (Modale Hilfsverben)

Modale Hilfsverben werden mit anderen Verben benutzt, um die Bedeutung des (Haupt-)Verbs (lexical verb) zu verändern. Das Hilfsverb steht im Englischen immer vor dem Hauptverb.

Grammar

I go to Amsterdam today. *go* = lexical verb
I must go to Amsterdam today *must* = auxiliary

Durch die Verwendung von „*must*" wird ein Element der Verpflichtung/Notwendigkeit dem Verb hinzugefügt, wodurch eine andere Bedeutung entsteht. Modale Hilfsverben sind:

can   could   may   might   must   need   ought   shall   should   will   would

Beispielsätze mit modalen Hilfsverben:

1. Vorhersage: *will/shall*
   We *will* all *be gone* in a hundred years.
   In hundert Jahren sind wir alle nicht mehr da.

2. Willensäußerung: *will/shall*
   I *shall look after* them.
   Ich werde für sie sorgen.

3. Bereitschaft/Wunsch: *will/would/shall*
   Would you *help* me to undress him?
   Würden Sie mir helfen, ihn auszuziehen?

4. In der Lage sein zu: *can/could*
   She *could do* it by herself if she had to.
   Sie könnte es alleine tun, wenn es nötig wäre.

5. Zustimmung: *can/may*
   Can I *have* a drink of water?
   Darf ich um einen Schluck Wasser bitten?

6. Unterstellung/nicht wirklich: *would*
I *would love to* work with children.　　Ich würde gerne mit Kindern arbeiten.

7. Möglichkeit: *may/might* (vielleicht/ziemlich sicher)
She *may go* home tomorrow.　　Vielleicht darf sie morgen nach Hause.
She *might go* home tomorrow.　　Ziemlich sicher geht sie morgen nach Hause.

8. Sicherheit/Überzeugung: *must*
This man *must be* at least 98.　　Dieser Mann ist mindestens 98 Jahre alt.

9. Verpflichtung/Notwendigkeit: *must/need (to)*
You *must/need to go* and see a doctor.　　Sie müssen zu einem Arzt.
Aber:
You *need not* = Du musst nicht/es ist nicht nötig
You *must not* = Du darfst nicht

10. Wünschenswert: *should/ought to*
You *should go* home when you don't feel well.　　Sie sollten lieber nach Hause gehen, wenn Sie sich nicht wohl fühlen.

11. Wahrscheinlichkeit: *should/ought to*
The handover *ought to start* in 5 minutes.　　Die Übergabe muss in 5 Minuten beginnen.

Fill in the modal auxiliaries that fit.

Exercise

1. _____ I go now?
(Kann ich/darf ich jetzt gehen?)

2. If you hurry up, he _____ still be there.
(Wenn du dich beeilst, kannst du ihn vielleicht noch erwischen.)

3. We _____ tell him what happened.
(Wir müssen ihm erzählen, was passiert ist.)

4. It _____ be busy tomorrow.
(Vielleicht ist morgen viel los.)

5. You _____ fight against your disease.
(Sie müssen gegen die Krankheit kämpfen.)

6. We _____ start the immunization scheme tomorrow.
(Wir werden morgen mit dem Impfprogramm beginnen.)

7. The new ampoules _____ be delivered at 5.
(Wir erwarten die neuen Ampullen um 5.00 Uhr.)

8. You _____ set the villagers a good example.
(Sie müssen den Dorfbewohnern ein gutes Vorbild sein.)

9. We _____ never know what caused his death.
(Wir werden nie wissen, woran er gestorben ist.)

10. He _____ be old but he is still very strong.
(Er ist vielleicht alt, aber er ist immer noch sehr stark.)

5.5 Translation

Translate the following sentences.

1. Ich werde Sie schnellstens aufsuchen.

Exercise

_____

2. Sie sollten besser aufpassen.

_____

3. Sie dürfen weg, sobald Sie fertig sind.

_____

4. Sie müssen vorsichtiger sein.

_____

5. Können Sie für mich auf das Knöpfchen drücken?

_____

5.6 Preventative Medicine Statements

Are the following statements true or false?

	true	false	Exercise
1. A _screening_ is a number of check-ups in a school or clinic to look for early signs of illness.	❑	❑	
2. Babies are never screened to make sure their hips are not _dislocated_.	❑	❑	
3. Another name for _rubella_ is _German measles._	❑	❑	

4. A *puncher* is an apparatus with a lot of small needles used for immunization. ❏ ❏

5. A *cholera vaccination* is administered before the age of 1. ❏ ❏

6. It is not uncommon to give pregnant women a booster injection with the *tetanus vaccine.* ❏ ❏

7. People cannot become immune to a disease by giving ready-made *antibodies* extracted from other people. ❏ ❏

8. Polio vaccine or *Sabin* is often administered orally. ❏ ❏

9. *Rabies* is transmitted by mosquitoes. ❏ ❏

10. *Hib vaccine* gives protection against *Haemophilus influenzae* type B. ❏ ❏

5.7 Help Educate Parents in Child Nutrition

Text

1 Young children are taller and healthier than they were 30 years ago, but they still need to consume a more balanced diet, the biggest-ever survey of diet and nutrition in one-to-four-year-olds has found.

5 The National Diet and Nutrition Survey, commissioned jointly by the DoH and the Ministry of Agriculture, Fisheries and Foods, shows that while most pre-school children are getting the nutrients they need, one in 12 is anaemic, half are not getting recommended levels of vitamin A and most are consuming too much sugar and salt.

15 At the launch of the report this week the government urged health visitors, nurses and all those involved in educating parents on child nutrition to take note of the findings.

20 Health officials reiterated the need for children to eat meat once a week, increase consumption of fruit and vegetables and reduce the intake of confectionary and sweet fizzy drinks, particularly at bedtime. [...]

25 Jeremy Metters, the government's deputy chief medical officer, said at the launch of the report that the results of the survey were generally reassuring. 'Children are taller than they were in late 1960s, sug-

30 gesting that they are getting the right nutritional intake,' he said.

But he added that iron deficiency was a problem, with 84% of children under four having iron levels below the recommended levels. He said that there was also concern about the high levels of non-milk extrinsic sugars consumed, particularly those commonly found in confectionary and sweet fizzy drinks, because of the effect on dental health.

The survey showed that almost a quarter of children had night-time drinks that contained sugar, such as fruit squashes, and a higher proportion of children who had a bedtime drink had some tooth decay.

Dr Metters said the report contained a lot of messages for health visitors, nurses and GPS to inform patients about diet, but, at the end of the day, control lay with the parents.

He added: 'We can't knock on everyone's door. We can only offer advice. I don't think anyone would wish to deprive children of treats of sugar or chocolate. We are talking here about a question of balance and that balance is not in the right place.'

Quelle: *Nursing Times*, 1995; 91 (13).

Translate the following words to be found in the text above.   *Exercise*

1. _____ Eisenmangel

2. _____ gemeinsam

3. _____ Nährstoffe

4. _____ informieren

5. _____ Ministerium für Volksgesundheit

6. _____ schließlich

7. _____ Aufmerksamkeit schenken

8. _____ wiederholen

9. _____ Landwirtschaftsministerium

10. _____ im Auftrag von

11. _____ anämisch

12. _____ ausgeglichen

13. _____ genutzt

14. _____ ruhig stellend

15. _____ Süßigkeiten

16. _____ Karies

17. _____ Besorgnis

18. _____ Brauselimonade

19. _____ Untersuchung

20. _____ verwehren

5.8 Differences Between American English and British English

Information German words can often be translated into English in different ways. One of the factors that determine the translation is whether it is a British or American variation. Sometimes only the spelling differs, for example: colour (British English; BE) and color (American English; AE). However, in some occasions the word is different, for example: ill (BE) and sick (AE).

Exercise Fill in the gaps, using the words below.

closet flavour cheque Kinderwagen Krankengeld centre mean null traineeship diaper Programm Ehre ground floor Universität flashlight orthopaedist check orthopedist spilt holiday gerochen elevator vacation barf neighbours gynecologist neighbors mad Abfalleimer haematology behavior

	British English	American English
different words		
1. Erdgeschoss	_____	first floor
2. gemein	nasty	_____
3. Schrank	cupboard	_____
4. _____	pram	baby carriage
5. erbrechen	puke	_____
6. böse	angry	_____
7. Lift	lift	_____
8. Windel	nappy	_____
9. _____	nil/0	zero
10. Praktikum	_____	internship
11. _____	university	college/university
12. Ferien	_____	_____
13. _____	dustbin	garbage can
14. Taschenlampe	torch	_____
15. _____	sickness benefit	sick-pay

16. Nachbarn _____ _____

17. Zentrum _____ center

18. Scheck _____ _____

19. _____ honour honor

20. verschüttet _____ spilled

21. _____ smelt smelled

22. Gynäkologe gynaecologist _____

23. Hämatologie _____ hematology

24. Orthopäde _____ _____

25. _____ programme program

26. Geschmack _____ flavor

27. Verhalten behaviour _____

5.9 Disease Prevention

Try to fit the following definitions into the diagram.

Puzzle

1. Other name for vitamin B2.
2. Common 'place' for injection.
3. Best food for a baby.
4. Metallic element essential to life especially for the proper functioning of muscle and nervous tissue. Symbol is Mg.
5. The rate at which a disease happens or exists.
6. Loss or deficiency of water in body tissues.
7. Cleanliness.
8. Often used for oral administration of polio vaccine.

9. A poison produced by a living organism.
10. An additional amount of a drug to strengthen the effect of some of the same drug that was given earlier.
11. The production of immunity by artificial means.
12. … is better than wealth.
13. Any substance that the body regards as foreign or potentially dangerous and against which it produces antibodies.
14. Fundamental constituents of all proteins.
15. One of a group of structurally related proteins that act as antibodies.

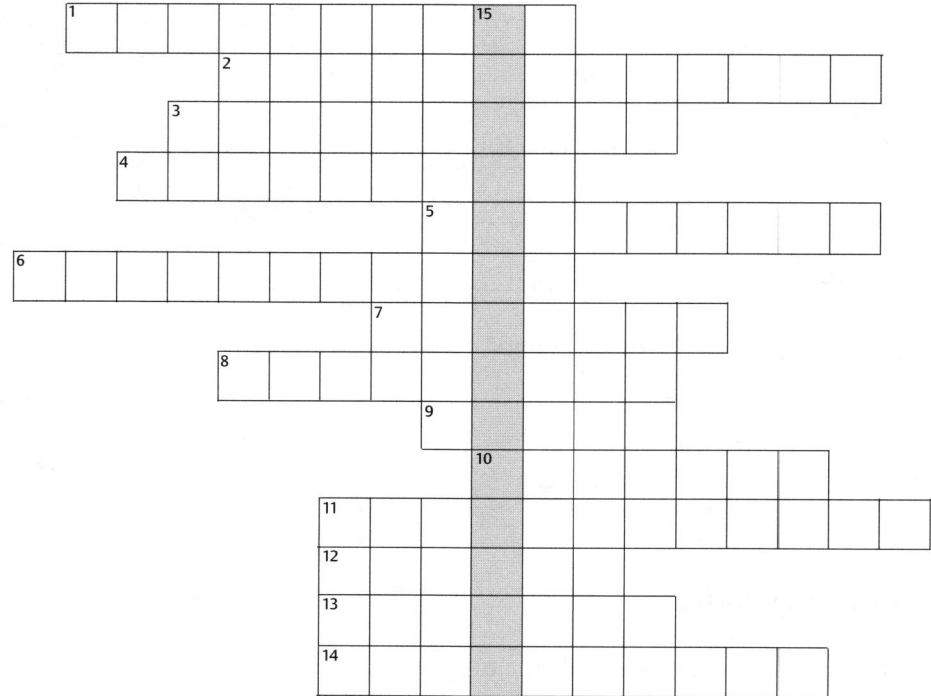

Treating Illness

6.1 'Dangerous' Medicine

Human insulin reality and myths

Text

An article in last week's Sunday Times linked the deaths of people with diabetes to the use of human insulin.

There is no evidence whatsoever to support this.

5 The British Diabetic Association (BDA) wants to reassure the very large number of people whom may have been caused stress by the contents of this article.
Dr Matthew Kiln was quoted as saying of 10 human insulin: 'Some have died because of it.' This comment cannot be backed up by evidence.
200,000 people use human insulin. Imagine how they felt when they read what 15 this doctor had to say. Imagine the unnecessary fear this comment could cause to many thousands of people who use human insulin without such problems.
The unexpected deaths of people with di-20 abetes, especially the young, is a tragic, serious and disturbing problem. These deaths have occurred over several decades, well before the introduction of human insulin. Numbers of such deaths 25 have not risen since human insulin became available. Only thorough research can identify the true cause of these tragedies, so they can be avoided in the future.
30 The BDA is leading this research, looking at 30,000 people treated with insulin. This is expected to cast light on the true circumstances and causes of this long-term, unexplained problem. Until more is 35 known, irresponsible speculation can only be damaging to the people that mat-ter, those who live with diabetes.
The article claims that a study, presented earlier this week at the BDA's Medical and 40 Scientific Section meeting, suggested human insulin may be 'dangerous'. Dr Simon Heller, the study's principal author, has said that this study does not suggest that human insulin is dangerous. Once 45 again, hearsay is the source of such claims.
The BDA recognizes that a small, but significant, proportion of people using human insulin have had problems. Everyone 50 who uses insulin should have the right to use animal or human insulins, a right the BDA strongly supports.
The BDA's highly successful Insulin Campaign petition, which calls for the con-55 tinued availability of animal insulins, has attracted over 140,000 signatures from the diabetes community. The thrust of the Campaign is freedom of choice, so that people can use the insulin which 60 they believe suits them best.
Freedom of choice includes the right to use human insulin, which 85% of insulin users do. Ill-founded allegations, linking human insulin to deaths without a shred 65 of conclusive evidence, threaten the freedom of some 200,000 people who rely on this insulin and happily use it every day to stay alive. The choice of insulin should

be a joint decision between the health professional and the person with diabetes. The BDA supports all people with diabetes. There are over 1 million in total in the UK with both types of diabetes. This includes people using human insulin and animal insulin and, just as importantly, the majority of people with diabetes who control their condition without insulin. They all deserve the right to balanced and accurate information.

The BDA condemns any individual or organisation that unnecessarily causes distress to people with diabetes and those who care for them.

If you would like further information on insulin, or any other aspect of diabetes, please contact the BDA's Careline on 0171-6366221. The Careline operates between 9 am and 5 pm, Monday to Friday. You can also write to us at the address given below.

BRITISH DIABETIC ASSOCIATION
10 Queen Anne Street, London W1M OBD.
reg.Charity No. 215199.
A charity helping people with diabetes and supporting diabetes research.

Quelle: *The Observer,* 2-4-1995

Exercise

Try to answer the following questions about the text.

1. *linked* in line 2 means:
   a) to cause
   b) to arrange
   c) to connect
   d) to harm

2. *to reassure* in line 6 means:
   a) to insure
   b) to erase
   c) to explain
   d) to comfort

3. *backed up* in line 11 means:
   a) to support
   b) to go backwards
   c) to ignore
   d) to finish

4. *decade* in line 23 means:
   a) a period of 1000 years
   b) a period of 100 years
   c) a period of 5 years
   d) a period of 10 years

5. *to cast light on* in line 32 means:
   a) to help to explain
   b) to shine
   c) to speak about
   d) to lie about

6. *circumstances* in line 32/33 refer to:
   a) ideas
   b) coincidences
   c) combination of facts
   d) positions

7. *hearsay* in line 45 means:
   a) the sense of hearing
   b) accusations
   c) the things we hear
   d) things said rather than proved

8. *thrust* in line 57 means:
   a) the main meaning
   b) belief in honesty
   c) combined group of firms
   d) the reason

9. *ill-founded* in line 63 means:
   a) feeling ill
   b) factual
   c) not sustained by reasons/facts
   d) against a law or rule

10. *conclusive* in line 65 means:
   a) putting an end to doubt
   b) being in agreement
   c) false
   d) happen at the same time

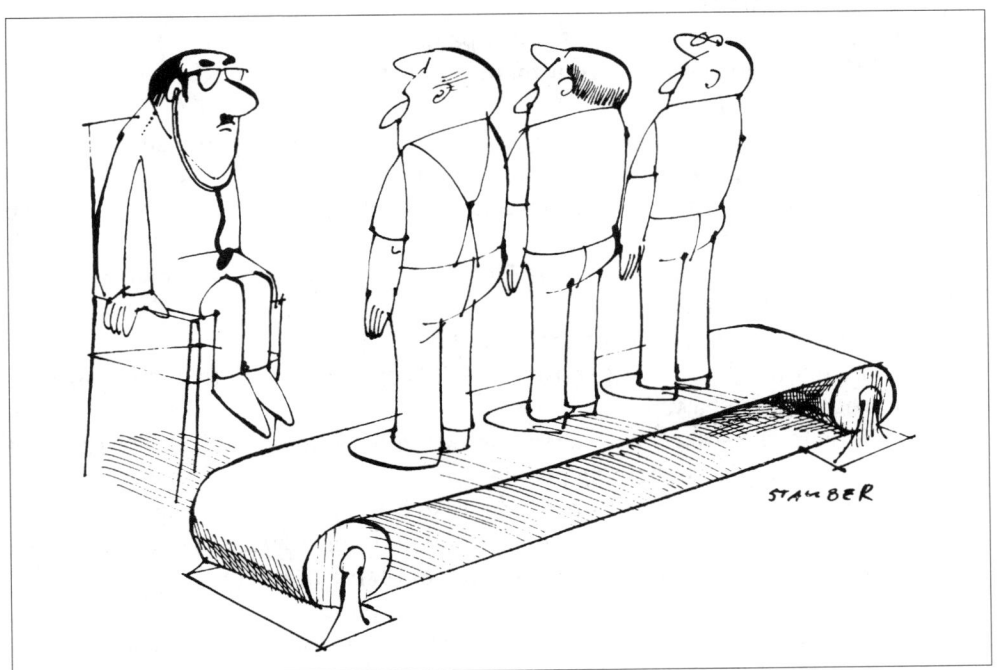

Quelle: Löwensteiner Cartoon Service (Hrsg.): Dr. med. Ironicus. Thieme, Stuttgart 1994 (S. 21)

6.2 Pains and Heartaches

Listen to the conversation between a patient, *Mr Yung (Mr Y)*, and two nurses, *Sharon (Sh) and Peter (P)*.

Conversation

Mr Y: Nurse, I can't sleep. I'm in such a pain.

Sh: Where does it hurt, Mr Yung?

Mr Y: All over the place. My belly, my back, my groin and even my legs are killing me.

Sh: Well, I'll give you one more sedative to settle down for the night but then you must really try to get some sleep.

Mr Y: All right, thanks, Sharon.
(*ten minutes later Peter enters the room*)

P: Are you still awake, Mr Yung?

Mr Y: I am indeed, oh nurse, I am sore all over. Can't you give me something to alleviate the pain?

P: Where does it bother you most?

Mr Y: It's these headaches, you know, and what about the stabbing pain in my chest? It won't stop either. It's driving me crazy. If I could only sleep for one hour and forget about these terrible pains!

P: All right, I'll go and check your medication chart.
(Peter returns after 5 minutes)
Mr Yung, what is going on here? Sharon has just given you a sedative. That was a very short while ago. Are you trying to pull my leg?

Mr Y: No, no I didn't mean to offend anyone but I really can't sleep, you must believe that. This is so embarrassing.

P: What is embarrassing, Mr Yung? Please try and tell me your problem.

Mr Y: Oh, it's the Mrs you see.

P: You mean your wife? What about her?

Mr Y: I miss her terribly, I can't get used to it. If I could only be with her. It's no good since she passed away.

P: Have you ever talked with someone of the bereavement services? They are usually very good in helping people.

Mr Y: What good will that do? Nobody wants to listen to a silly, grumpy old man.

P: Nonsense! What if I phone someone for you tomorrow and see how you feel about it after you've had a talk with one of their counsellors?

Mr Y: If you think that would help me, I might as well try.

P: That's the spirit! And what if I made you a hot drink now, maybe that will make you fall asleep?

Mr Y: Oh, yes, I wouldn't mind some hot milk, thank you.

P: I'll be back in a sec.
(when Peter returns with the milk Mr Yung is soundly asleep)

Exercise

Match the words from the conversation with their German counterparts. You cannot use all German words!

1. heartache	... **a)** Kopfschmerzen	... **j)** straucheln lassen
2. groins	... **b)** jemanden auf den	... **k)** Leisten
3. to alleviate	Arm nehmen	... **l)** lindern
4. to bother	... **c)** sterben	... **m)** schnarchend
5. to pull a person's leg	... **d)** weggehen	... **n)** kränken
6. to offend	... **e)** Reue	... **o)** schlimm
7. embarrassing	... **f)** Achselhöhlen	... **p)** fest
8. to pass away	... **g)** Kummer	... **q)** anfechten
9. bereavement	... **h)** stoppen	... **r)** peinlich
10. soundly	... **i)** belästigen	... **s)** Trauerfall
		... **t)** Gesäß

6.3 Medication

One of the important tasks of a nurse is to administer drugs and observe and control their effect. Most drugs are synthetic: they are produced in laboratories. They are based on substances contained in plants and herbs which have healing properties. Names for drugs are not always the same in every country, even when the product referred to contains the same substances. Nurses working abroad should be very aware of this!

Information

Study this medication information and say whether the following statements are true or false.

Exercise

Important information, read carefully!

Isoptin® SR 240mg

Active drug substance: verapamil hydrochloride

Film coated tablets with prolonged action
Calcium antagonist for the treatment of hypertension

Composition
1 film coated tablet contains 240 mg of verapamil hydrochloride.

Mode of action
The calcium antagonist verapamil inhibits the transmembrane influx of calcium ions into the heart and vascular smooth muscle cell. The antihypertensive effect of Isoptin stems from a decrease in peripheral vascular resistance — without an increase in heart rate as a reflex response. As early as day 1 of treatment blood pressure falls; the effect is found to persist also in long-term therapy. Isoptin is suitable for the treatment of all types of hypertension: for monotherapy in mild to moderate hypertension, combined with other hypertensives — in particular with diuretics and, according to more recent findings, with ACE inhibitors — in more severe types of hypertension.
Due to the calcium-antagonistic effect on the smooth vascular muscles of the coronaries, Isoptin enhances myocardial blood flow, even in poststenotic areas, and relieves coronary spasms.
Isoptin has a marked antiarrhythmic effect, particularly in supraventricular arrhythmias. It delays impulse conduction in the AV node. Owing to this, sinus rhythm is restored and/or ventricular rate is normalized, depending on the type of arrhythmia.

Indications
Hypertension.

Dosage and mode of administration
The doses of Isoptin SR 240 mg, individualized according to the severity of the disease, are to be taken regularly as prescribed by the physician. The film coated tablets are to be swallowed whole with some liquid, preferably with or shortly after meals.
Unless otherwise instructed, the daily dose for adults is 1 film coated tablet in the morning (patients requiring particularly gradual blood pressure lowering should be started on half a tablet taken in the morning). If after about 2 weeks of treatment a dose increase is found to be necessary the dose can be raised to a maximum of 2 film coated tablets daily (additionally 1 half to 1 film coated tablet in the evening after an interval of about 12 hours).
On long-term treatment a daily dose of 480 mg should not be exceeded; short-term dose increases are possible only when directed by the physician.
For children and adults requiring smaller doses of verapamil, Isoptin 40 mg and 80 mg are available.
In patients with impaired hepatic function the effect of verapamil is intensified and prolonged depending on the severity of the liver disease due to diminished drug metabolism. In these cases dosage should be adjusted with special care starting with low doses (e. g. in patients with hepatic cirrhosis with 1 tablet of Isoptin 40 mg 2—3 times daily).

Contraindications
Isoptin SR 240 mg should not be given in the following cases:
Cardiovascular shock, complicated acute myocardial infarction (bradycardia, marked hypotension, left ventricular failure), severe conduction disorders (2nd and 3rd degree AV block, sinoatrial block) and sick sinus syndrome (bradycardia-tachycardia syndrome).

Side effects
Particularly when given in high doses or in the presence of previous damage, some cardiovascular effects of verapamil may occasionally be greater than therapeutically desired: bradycardic arrthythmias, such as sinus bradycardia, sinus arrest with asystole, 2nd and 3rd degree AV block or bradyarrhythmia in atrial fibrillation, hypotension, development or aggravation of heart failure. Constipation has been reported frequently.
In rare cases nausea, vertigo or dizziness, headache, flushing, fatigue, nervousness, ankle oedemas, erythromelalgia and paraesthesia may occur. In very rare cases, there may be myalgia and arthralgia.
Single cases of allergic skin reactions (exanthema, pruritus, urticaria, angioneurotic oedema, Stevens-Johnson syndrome) have been reported, in addition to a reversible increase of trans-aminases and/or alkaline phosphatase, which is probably a sign of allergic hepatitis.
In very rare cases gynaecomastia, which so far has been fully reversible in all cases following discontinuation of the drug, has been observed in elderly patients under long-term treatment. Rises in prolactin levels have been reported.
On extremely rare occasions gingival hyperplasia, which is fully reversible when the drug is discontinued, may occur under long-term treatment.

Interactions
The simultaneous administration of Isoptin SR 240 mg and cardioactive drugs (e. g. betareceptor blockers, antiarrhythmics) or inhalation anaesthetics may lead to a mutual enhancement of the cardiovascular effects (AV blockade, bradycardia, hypotension, heart failure). When given in combination with quinidine in patients with hypertrophic obstructive cardiomyopathy single cases of hypotension and pulmonary oedema were observed. Intravenous betareceptor blockers should not be given to patients under treatment with Isoptin SR 240 mg.
Isoptin SR 240 mg may intensify the blood pressure-lowering effect of other antihypertensives.
Rises in digoxin plasma levels under concomitant administration of verapamil have been reported. Physicians should be on the alert for symptoms of possible digoxin toxicity. The digitalis level should be determined and the glycoside dose reduced; if required.
There have also been occasional reports on interactions with carbamazepine (potentiated by verapamil, neurotoxic side effects), lithium (attenuated by verapamil, enhanced neurotoxicity), cyclosporin, theophylline, (rise of plasma level by verapamil), rifampicin, phenytoin and phenobarbital (reduced plasma level and effects of verapamil attenuated). Verapamil plasma levels may be increased under concomitant administration of cimetidine. The effect of muscle relaxants may be potentiated.

Precautions
When treating hypertension with Isoptin SR 240 mg, monitoring of the patient's blood pressure at regular intervals is required. Depending on individual susceptibility, the patient's ability to drive a vehicle or operate machinery may be impaired. This is particularly true in the initial stages of treatment, when changing over from another drug, and also with respect to the consumption of alcohol.
Care should be taken in:
1st degree AV block, bradycardia < 50 beats/min, hypotension < 90 mmHg systolic pressure, atrial fibrillation/flutter and simultaneous pre-excitation syndrome, e. g. WPW syndrome (risk of inducing ventricular tachycardia), heart failure (compensation with cardiac glycosides, for example, before initiating treatment).
Isoptin SR 240 mg should not be given during pregnancy (especially in the first trimester) and lactation unless, in the physician's judgement, it is essential for the patient's well-being.

Expiry date
Do not use beyond the expiry date indicated on the carton.

Trade packs
20 film coated tablets.

Other forms
Trade packs containing 50 and 100 tablets of Isoptin 40 mg.
Trade packs containing 20 and 50 tablets of Isoptin 80 mg.
Trade packs containing 20 tablets of Isoptin 120 mg.
Trade packs containing 20 tablets of Isoptin retard.
Trade packs containing 5 ampoules, 2 ml each (5 mg of verapamil hydrochloride/2 ml).

Store the drug carefully!
Keep out of the reach of children!

Knoll AG · D-67008 Ludwigshafen · Germany   **knoll**

---

		true	false
1.	Isoptin is used for the treatment of hypertension.	❏	❏
2.	The tablets have to be chewed thoroughly.	❏	❏
3.	The normal dosage of this medicine is 480 mg 2–3 times daily.	❏	❏
4.	One of the side effects of this drug is low blood pressure.	❏	❏

5. Patients using this drug often complain of diarrhoea.   ❏   ❏

6. When patients are using this dosage of Isoptin their blood pressure should be checked regularly.   ❏   ❏

7. Driving is not influenced by this drug.   ❏   ❏

8. In the first three months pregnant women can use this drug.   ❏   ❏

9. When a woman is breast-feeding she should not use this drug.   ❏   ❏

10. This drug can also be injected.   ❏   ❏

6.4 English-German Equivalents

Exercise

Drugs are available in different forms. Match the English words with their German translations.

1. tablet		**a)**	Injektionsflüssigkeit
2. coated tablet		**b)**	Tablette
3. granules		**c)**	Mixtur
4. cream		**d)**	Tropfenflüssigkeit
5. elixir		**e)**	Hustensirup
6. powder		**f)**	Dragee
7. capsule		**g)**	Creme
8. mixture		**h)**	Gurgelflüssigkeit
9. lozenge ['lazɪndʒ]		**i)**	Salbe
10. solution for injection		**j)**	Fett
11. ointment		**k)**	Kapsel
12. liniment		**l)**	Balsam
13. balsam		**m)**	Hustentablette
14. suppository		**n)**	Lotion
15. lotion		**o)**	Tinktur, Auszug
16. gargle		**p)**	Inhalation
17. inhalation		**q)**	Spray
18. spray		**r)**	Stuhlgangzäpfchen
19. drops		**s)**	Granulat
20. linctus		**t)**	Puder

6.5 The Plural (Mehrzahl)

Grammar

Regelmäßige Substantive erhalten im Englischen für die Pluralform meistens ein „*s*", z.B.: nurse – nurses, oder ein „*es*", wenn sie auf einen Zischlaut enden, z.B.: box – boxes.

1. Beispiele für *unregelmäßige* Pluralformen:
calf	calves
life	lives
self	selves
wife	wives

2. Veränderung von Selbstlauten
foot	feet
man	men
tooth	teeth
woman	women

3. Veränderung nach Mitlauten + y
country	countries
lady	ladies

4. Einige Wörter erhalten ein „-en"
child	children

5. Einige Wörter bleiben gleich
   Chinese
   means
   species

6. Lateinische Wörter: einige (*) haben zwei Pluralformen
focus*	focuses/foci
formula	formulae
radius*	radiuses/radii
syllabus*	syllabuses/syllabi
vertebra	vertebrae

7. Einige griechische Wörter
analysis	analyses
basis	bases
criterion	criteria
phenomenon	phenomena
thesis	theses

8. Einige Wörter existieren nur im Singular
   abuse
   information
   progress

9. Einige Wörter existieren nur im Plural
contents
scissors
tights
physics
wages

Exercise

Fill in the correct plural.

1. How many _____ did you bring? (Pyjamas)

2. He is looking for his _____. (Brille)

3. The child lost two of her _____. (Zähne)

4. They should eat more _____. (Kartoffeln)

5. Where did the _____ go to? (Krankenhausbusse)

6. Five _____ went for an operation today. (Frauen)

7. I will hand out the _____ at noon. (Arzneimittel)

8. You'll have to accept her _____. (Auffassungen)

9. Two _____ fell out. (Planken/Bohlen)

10. He had two _____ today. (Bäder)

6.6 Translation

Exercise

Translate the following sentences.

1. Ich kann die Schere nicht finden.

_____

2. Die Patienten haben wenig Forderungen gestellt.

_____

3. Sie ließ zwei Messer fallen.

_____

4. Die Analyse verwendet drei Kriterien.

_____

5. Können Sie diese Damen in ihr Zimmer bringen?

_____

6.7 Fluency: Care plans

Find a partner and pick one of the care plans below. Pretend you are in a meeting in which the patient's care will be discussed. Without looking at them can you come up with the actions mentioned in the care plans. Your partner is allowed to assist you. Swap roles when discussing the different care plans.

Exercise

D. 21 Care plan 7

Date	no.	PROBLEM / NEED	EXPECTED OUTCOME	evaluation time date
		_____ is dehydrated	Relieve symptoms within	
		or a risk of dehydration	48 hours.	
			Maintain hydration.	
			Safely & correctly maintain IVI.	

D. 21 Care plan 7

ACTION	date sign	EVALUATION	date sign
1. Assess patient for signs of confusion,			
dry skin or dry mucosa			
2. Maintain accurate fluid balance.			
3. Ensure IV fluid rota is maintained.			
4. Ensure giving set is changed every 72 hours.			
5. Encourage oral fluids.			
6. Observe for signs of fluid overload:			
a) breathlessness.			
b) oedema.			
7. Encourage oral care.			

D. 21 Care plan 8

Date	no.	PROBLEM / NEED	EXPECTED OUTCOME	evaluation time date
		_____ has unstable	Maintain safety at all times.	
		blood sugars.		
			Monitor & return blood sugars to	
			within normal limits.	

D. 21 Care plan 8

ACTION	date sign	EVALUATION	date sign
1. Monitor blood sugars as directed			
i.e. 1 – 6 hourly.			
2. Administer sliding scale insulin / IVI as			
prescribed			
3. Urinalysis for glucose & ke tones.			
(Daily or if BM over 20 mmols)			
4. Monitor TPR 6 hourly.			
5. Observe for physical signs of hypo or			
hyperglycaemia			
e.g. sweating, confusion, agitation,			
drowsiness, pear drop halitosis.			
6. Observe fluid balance.			
7. Provide diabetic diet.			
8. Inform medical staff of any abnormalities.			
9. Refer to diabetes centre if necessary			
for education			
10. Explain all nursing procedures to			
patient & relatives.			

Care Plan for Patients Short of Breath

Date	no.	PROBLEM / NEED	EXPECTED OUTCOME	evaluation time date
		_____ is	Relieve symptoms &	
		short of breath.	promote comfort.	
			Monitor condition.	

Care Plan for Patients Short of Breath

ACTION	date sign	EVALUATION	date sign
1. Observe respiratory rate, depth & rhythm _____ hrly.			
2. Observe _____ colour for cyanosis or pallor.			
3. Record TP BP _____ hrly.			
4. Encourage expectoration note, colour, amount obtain a specimen.			
5. Provide sputum pot & tissues.			
6. Refer to physiotherapy.			
7. Nurse upright & support with pillows.			
8. Note any increasing anxiousness, restlessness or confusion.			
9. Administer oxygen as prescribed.			
10. Give medication as prescribed.			
11. Monitor effectiveness via pre & post nebuliser peak flows.			
12. Encourage a good standard of oral hygiene.			
13. Refer to respiratory nurse if applicable to undergo teaching.			

D. 21 Care plan 14

Date	no.	PROBLEM / NEED	EXPECTED OUTCOME	evaluation time date
		_____ has a	Maintain safety monitor	
		head injury.	condition for complication.	

D. 21 Care plan 14

ACTION	date sign	EVALUATION	date sign
1. Baseline observations TPR BP			
2. Assess _____ state of			
conscious level using the Glasgow coma scale.			
Note if orietated in time, place & person.			
3. Observe pupils reaction to light, size &			
any compared differences in each side.			
4. Observe for loss of sensation or power			
in limbs			
5. Monitor for headache, note position,			
severity & duration. Administer analgesia			
prn if prescribed & note its effectiveness.			
6. Note any visual / speech disturbances or			
confusion			
7. Observe for nausea or vomiting.			
8. Repeat neurological observations as per			
chart _____hourly.			
9. Note head wound if any, position, size,			
sutures, discharge. Apply sterile dressing			
10. Observe for any discharge (clear watery			
fluid or blood) from ears or nose.			
11. Advise patient to remain on bedrest.			
12. Offer reassurance and explanations to			
patient & relatives			

D. 21 Care plan 11

Date	no.	PROBLEM / NEED	EXPECTED OUTCOME	evaluation time date
		_____ is experiencing	To relieve symptoms an treat	
		chest pain and	cause	
		breathlessness		

D. 21 Care plan 11

ACTION	date sign	EVALUATION	date sign
1. Observe respiratory rate _____hrly.			
2. Observe for cyanosis, administer oxygen as prescribed and monitor effects.			
3. Record oxygen saturations _____ hourly as required.			
4. Encourage limited activities and bed rest.			
5. Administer intravenous heparin as prescribed, ensure pump is working correctly and set at the correct rate.			
6. Give analgesia as prescribed and monitor effects.			
7. Record blood pressure, pulse and temperature _____ hourly.			
8. Explain all procedures and investigations to patient.			
9. Provide ted stockings and encourage their use, with a daily two hour removal rest period.			
10. Encourage _____ to report further symptoms such as pain and swelling il legs.			
11. Assist with activities restricted due to condition and bed rest.			

ACTION	date sign	EVALUATION	date sign
12. Explain control of anti coagulants when			
commenced on warfarin and the impor-tance			
of the anti coagulant clinic.			
13. Report any abnormalities to medical staff.			

6.8 Operating Theatre

The following picture shows an operating theatre. What is what?

Exercise

1. time-elapse clock
2. mask
3. rubber gloves
4. gown
5. cap
6. surgeon
7. anaesthesist
8. theatre nurse
9. electric knife
10. adjustable light
11. suture
12. gauzes
13. scalpel
14. forceps
15. surgical tweezers
16. non-crushing clamp
17. twin gastrointestinal clamp
18. abdominal retractor
19. bistoury

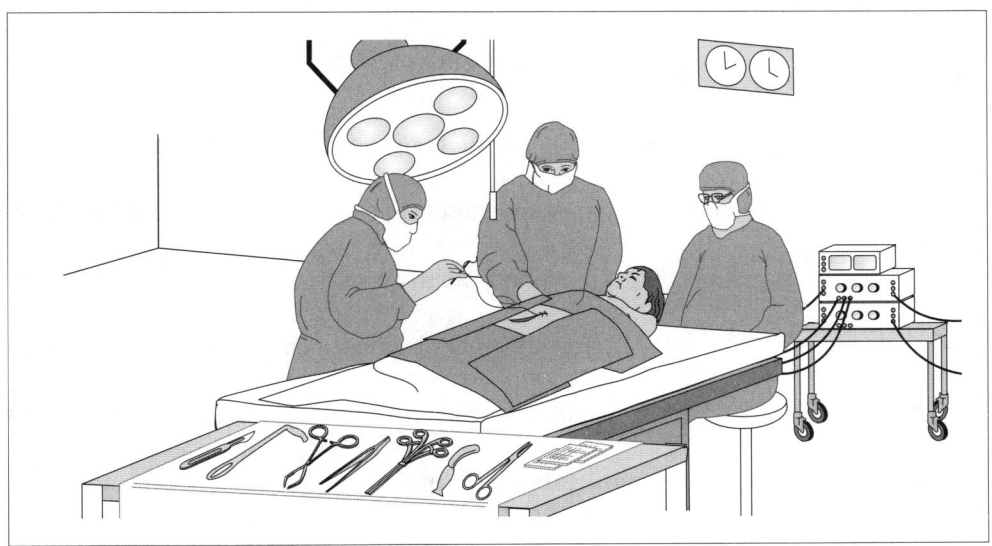

6.9 Different Operations and Treatments

Exercise

Choose the right definition of the following words.

1. amputation
2. acupuncture
3. colectomy
4. laryngectomy
5. chiropractic

6. oophorectomy
7. osteotomy
8. laparoscopy
9. chemotherapy
10. lithotripsy

... **a)** Partial or total removal of the larynx by surgery.

... **b)** The manual movement of the vertebrae to relieve the effect of subluxating transverse processes on the nerve roots.

... **c)** Insertion of needles into particular parts of the body for treatment of disease or relief of pain.

... **d)** Special combination of drugs that arrest the progress of, or eradicate disease without causing irreversible injury to healthy tissues.

... **e)** The treatment of choice for a patient who has renal calculus.

... **f)** Excision of the colon.

... **g)** Synonymous with ovariectomy which refers to excision of an ovary.

... **h)** To cut a bone into two parts, followed by realignment of the ends to allow healing.

... **i)** The removal of a limb, part of a limb, or any other portion of the body.

... **j)** Endoscopic examination of the pelvic organs by the transperitoneal route.

6.10 Treating Illness

Exercise

Fill in the gaps with the words below.

All (1) _____ act differently on the body. For this reason some have to be taken after a meal and others on an empty stomach; some need to be mixed with water and others (2) _____ whole. The (3) _____ retain an important place in the treatment of gastrointestinal diseases such as dyspepsia, peptic ulcer and (4) _____. Some drugs are given as a prophylactic. Patients who are at risk of embolisation are often treated with oral (5) _____. Some medicines cause side-effects or (6) _____. The doctor has to weigh the advantages against the disadvantages when (7) _____ medicines. Sometimes people refuse treatments because of their religion. (8) _____, for example, strongly object to the infusion of (9) _____. Without their (10) _____ transfusion cannot take place.

*blood   antacids   consent   anticoagulants   medicines   gastritis   Jehovah's Witnesses
swallowed   prescribing   allergic reactions*

Unit 7   Obstetrics and Neonates

7.1 Legislation and Reproductive Technology

Text

IVF surrogacy

1 The prohibition of IVF surrogacy in Victoria is an example of inappropriate regulation by statute legislation. IVF surrogacy is a procedure used by a woman who has no
5 functional uterus, but can provide eggs to form an IVF embryo that will be transferred to a surrogate. Surrogacy itself is not illegal in Victoria, provided that no advertising, payment or legal contracts
10 are made. However, a section of the Infertility (Medical Procedures) Act relating to the use of donor eggs stipulates that embryos are not to be transferred to a recipient unless she is 'unlikely to become
15 pregnant as a result of a procedure other than a procedure to which this Act applies'. This requirement inadvertently outlaws IVF surrogacy. For strictly legal purposes, a potential surrogate must be
20 infertile, with total ovarian failure, although for clinical purposes she must be potentially fertile! This ruling is an example of dangerous and ambiguous 'quickdraw' legislation that was accurately pre-
25 dicted by Justice Michael Kirby in 1985.
A further difficulty with IVF surrogacy occurs because the Status of Children (Amendment) Act 1984 (Vic.) states that the woman who gives birth is the mother
30 of the child for all legal purposes. This Act was specifically introduced to establish legal motherhood for an infertile woman conceiving through the donor oocyte program, and has been of immense value in
35 this context. The surrogate situation, however, requires a reversal of roles. A simple amendment to this Act could accommodate the few cases of IVF surrogacy requested by infertile couples in Aus-
40 tralia each year.
In 1988 the newly established National Bioethics Consultative Committee (NBCC), consisting of 13 experts from around Australia, investigated all aspects of surroga-
45 cy and gave much attention to the ethical principles underlying the debate. The NBCC concluded that surrogacy arrangements should be allowed under strict control with uniform national Australian
50 legislation. Both federal and State health ministers unanimously rejected these recommendations, preferring instead to maintain the status quo, in which conflicting State legislation effectively re-
55 stricts infertile couples from receiving IVF surrogacy in Australia, compelling them to travel overseas for this treatment. This approach is at variance with the conclusions of the NBCC and with society's atti-
60 tude to surrogacy. The Morgan Gallup poll in April 1994 also showed 52.7% of Australians approved of altruistic surrogacy, in which no payment is made to the surrogate.

Quelle: *The Medical Journal of Australia* 1995; 163:205.

Translate the following words from the text.

1. legislation (l. 3)	..... **a)**	Gesetz
2. surrogacy (l. 7)	..... **b)**	unabsichtlich
3. act (l. 11)	..... **c)**	undeutlich
4. stipulates (l. 12)	..... **d)**	Eizelle zur Bildung des 1. Polkörpers
5. recipient (l. 13/14)	..... **e)**	Richter
6. inadvertently (l. 17)	..... **f)**	gleichlautend
7. outlaws (l. 18)	..... **g)**	Empfehlungen
8. infertile (l. 20)	..... **h)**	Leihmutterschaft
9. ambiguous (l. 23)	..... **i)**	helfen
10. Justice (l. 25)	..... **j)**	unfruchtbar
11. legal purposes (l. 30)	..... **k)**	unveränderter Zustand
12. oocyte (l. 33)	..... **l)**	Gesetzgebung
13. reversal (l. 36)	..... **m)**	Empfänger
14. accommodate (l. 37/38)	..... **n)**	im Gegensatz zu
15. uniform (l. 49)	..... **o)**	gesetzliche Aspekte
16. unanimously (l. 51)	..... **p)**	verbieten
17. recommendations (l. 52)	..... **q)**	bestimmt
18. status quo (l. 53)	..... **r)**	selbstlos
19. at variance with (l. 58)	..... **s)**	einhellig
20. altruistic (l. 62)	..... **t)**	Revision

7.2 The Unplanned Hospital Visit

Listen to the conversation between a *nurse (N), Ms Roefs (R)* and *Ms Michen (M)*.

N: How are you feeling this morning, Ms Roefs? Did you sleep well?

R: I did not! I can't sleep, I can't eat, I can't even move!
This is just not how I imagined it would be. I will be crippled for the rest of my life.

N: Well, I know it won't do you much good now, but I can assure you, you'll be feeling much better in a few days. I'll help you out of bed first.

R: Out of bed? Are you out of your mind? There's no way I'm getting out of this bed. Just leave me in peace and come back next month or so.

M: It will do you much good, Anne-Mary; you should really try it. Part of the pain is probably caused by stiffness of your muscles. Get them moving again.

R: It's easy for you. You had it all planned, but I didn't want to go to hospital in the first place. If I can get my hands on those midwives. I still can't believe they never noticed it was a breech presentation. There must be someone who is smart enough to distinguish between a bum and a face.

N: Now, take a deep breath and I'll help you up. Try to relax your belly and don't put any pressure on the stitches from the Caesarean section. Take it easy, give me your drip.

M: Well done. Come and sit over here so we can have a chat and you can admire my twins before I go home.

R: No, I won't. I can't be bothered with your gossip. Why is everybody allowed to go home after a day or so except me? This whole business is so bloody unfair.

N: I'll bring your baby so you can start breast-feeding. He's so cute.

R: He! It's a she for heaven's sake and her name is Kay!

N: Oh, I'm awfully sorry, but I thought it was a...

R: It's a she and thank you nurse, I can manage on my own now.
(picks up her daughter)
Hello sunshine, how are you today?

Exercise   Answer the following questions

1. Why did Ms Michen give birth in hospital?

_____

2. Why is Ms Roefs complaining about her midwives?

_____

3. How is Ms Roefs' fluid intake taken care of?

_____

4. How did Ms Roefs give birth to her daughter?

_____

5. Is Kay bottle-fed?

_____

7.3 Labour and Delivery

Normal Delivery

Information   Labour usually starts 280 days after conception. There are three stages of labour and delivery.

1. *dilatation stage (USA dilation)*
   the muscular wall of the uterus begins contracting while the cervix expands. This may take 18-24 hours in the first pregnancy. The amnion ruptures, releasing amniotic fluid to the exterior. The degree of dilatation is measured by *vaginal examination.* Dilatation ends when the cervix is fully opened, which is approximately 10 cm.

2. *expulsion stage*
   the baby passes through the vagina, assisted by contractions of the abdominal muscles and pushing by the mother. The baby is assisted in delivery and rotated as the shoulders are presented. During delivery it may be necessary to enlarge the vaginal opening.
   This is done by a cut in the perineum: *episiotomy* [ə,pɪzɪ'atəmɪ]. Once the infant has been delivered the umbilical cord is cut.

3. *placental stage*
   the placenta and membranes are separated from the wall of the uterus and pushed downwards by pushing and contractions of the uterus.

Special Delivery

1. *expression*   *Information*
   Expulsion of the fetus or placenta by pressing with both hands on fundus of uterus.

2. *vacuum extraction*
   Delivery assisted by a suction device that is attached to the head of the fetus, after which traction is slowly applied.

3. *forceps delivery*
   When the baby is delivered by having its head held and pulled by (obstetrical) forceps.

4. *Caesarean section*
   A surgical operation in which the baby is delivered through an incision in the abdominal wall. When possible this incision will be transverse across the lowest and narrowest part of the abdomen (lower uterine segment); this is also referred to as a 'bikini cut'.

Translate the following words from the information above.

1. _____ Kaiserschnitt

2. _____ Wehen

3. _____ Befruchtung

4. _____ Öffnen des Muttermundes

5. _____ Zangengeburt

6. _____ Nabelschnur

7. _____ Fruchtblase

7.4 Relativpronomen

Grammar

Relativpronomen können verweisen auf Personen, Tiere und Sachen.
Die englischen Relativpronomen sind:

	Einzahl	*Mehrzahl*
who(m)	der, die, das, wer – das, was	die, welche
which	dito	dito
that	dito	dito
whose	dessen/wessen	deren
what	welches	welche
which	welches/dasjenige	welche/diejenigen

Im Englischen gelten folgende Regeln:

1. Für *Personen* benutzt man: *who, whom, whose.*

   Who als Subjekt des Satzes:
   Have you seen the baby *who* is sleeping in the incubator?
   That's the woman *who* had a miscarriage.

   Haben Sie das Baby gesehen, das im Inkubator schläft?
   Das ist die Frau, die eine Fehlgeburt hatte.

Whom als Akkusativobjekt. Nach einer Präposition ist *whom* bindend.

She is the doctor *who(m)* I spoke to earlier.	Sie ist die Ärztin, mit der ich früher gesprochen habe.
The girl *who(m)* I was talking to is a theatre nurse.	Das Mädchen, mit dem ich gesprochen habe, ist Operationsschwester.
Is that the girl to *whom* you gave the blanket?	Ist das das Mädchen, dem Sie die Decke gegeben haben?

Whose bei einem 2. Fall:

The man *whose* wife collapsed.	Der Mann, dessen Frau kollabierte.
Are you the midwife *whose* patient ran off?	Sind Sie die Hebamme, deren Patientin davongelaufen ist?

2. Für *Tiere* und *Dinge* benutzt man *which*

The crib *which* you see over there belongs to Danny.	Das Kinderbettchen, das Sie dort sehen, ist von Danny.
The dog *which* bit the child was put down.	Der Hund, der das Kind gebissen hat, wurde getötet.

In einschränkenden adjektivischen Nebensätzen (notwendige Hinzufügung) darf man:

3. *that* anstelle von *who* oder *which* benutzen

I don't like people *that/who* are indifferent.	Ich habe einen Widerwillen gegen gleichgültige Menschen.
I did not hear the news *that/which* was broadcast.	Ich habe die Nachrichten, die gesendet wurden, nicht gehört.

4. oder das Pronomen *weglassen;* dies darf jedoch nur dann erfolgen, wenn das Pronomen kein Subjekt ist und keine Präposition vorausgeht

The boy ( ) the drunken driver ran over, has just died.	Der Junge, der von dem betrunkenen Fahrer überfahren wurde, ist gerade gestorben.
Is Mary the manager *that/who* sacked you?	Ist Mary die Leiterin, die dich entlassen hat?

7.5 Translation

Exercise Translate the following sentences.

1. Dies ist das Mädchen, für das wir Arzneimittel fertig gemacht haben.

_____

2. Von wem ist die Windel?

_____

3. Ich ging zu der Hebamme, die Dienst hatte.

_____

4. Die Milch, die verdünnt wurde, roch muffig.

_____

5. Weißt Du, wer diesen Kinderwagen hier abgestellt hat?

_____

7.6 Staying Afloat: Water-Birth Practice

Text

Midwives have been warned that they need to look at their training and experience if they are to develop good practice in water-birthing.

A newly published study by the National Peri-natal Epidemiology Unit, Oxford, highlights the amount of work needed to establish the safety of water-births. It says that there is still no standardised data collection system in the NHS and midwives need to be auditing their practice on a national level.

Mary Renfrew, professor of midwifery at Leeds University, who headed the study, explains that its aim was to describe the extent of practice and availability of water-births in provider units. She says that safety would have to be addressed separately because thousands of women would need to be involved in such a trial. 'Many units have very small numbers of births where water is used and midwives need to be looking at where they are getting the training and experience to look after such women,' said Professor Renfrew. 'How are they learning and how are they setting up guidelines? What criteria are they using?' 'We were looking at the safety aspect but without knowing the extent of practice it is difficult to do a trial. What we show is that there is no evidence to stop the practice and what we need to do now is focus on the safety side.'

The study surveyed 219 heads of midwifery or equivalent post-holders. Labour in water had taken place in all provider units and 89% had pools, others used

baths. Some 8255 women had laboured
40 in the birthing pool or bath but got out for
the birth, while 4494 women gave birth
in the water. Figures were estimated and,
because of the retrospective nature of the
study, the researchers advise that the
45 data are treated with caution. [...] 'We
asked midwives directly about the number of problems for mothers and babies
and what we got were estimates.' [...]

'The message to midwives is that they
50 should be monitoring and auditing all
water-births. It is a new practice and
should be treated as such. Midwives need
to take care over training and experience
and set up guidelines which are sensitive
55 and take account of the best experience.'

Quelle: *Nursing Times* 1995; 19(16): 22.

Are the following statements about the text true or false?   *true*   *false*   *Exercise*

1. Information on water-birth is recorded in different ways.   ❏   ❏
2. Safety aspects need to be studied more thoroughly.   ❏   ❏
3. 8255 women had given birth in the birthing pool.   ❏   ❏
4. Midwives should edit all water-births.   ❏   ❏
5. Midwives could not give exact figures about the problems.   ❏   ❏

7.7 Postpartum and Neonatal Care

Choose the appropriate answer.   *Exercise*

1. In the postpartum period:
   a) amniocentesis is carried out
   b) the perineum and perineal pad are checked
   c) no noise is permitted
   d) the patient is put into a Sims' position

2. Red vaginal discharge is called:
   a) phenylketonuria
   b) colostrum
   c) amniotic fluid
   d) lochia

3. Involution is the:
   a) shrinking of uterus to its normal size after childbirth
   b) first secretion from the breast
   c) increase of the uterus
   d) premature separation of the placenta

4. Urine retention is indicated by:
   a) presence of episiotomy
   b) signs of inflammation
   c) fetal distress
   d) a uterus that is unusually high or pushed to one side

5. The neonate is evaluated by:
   a) the Apgar score
   b) a PKU test
   c) a gastric analysis (GA)
   d) an arterial blood gas study (ABG)

6. A premature baby is often nursed in a:
   a) perambulator
   b) incubator or isolette
   c) stockinette cap
   d) nursery

7. Babies who are jaundiced may be:
   a) circumcized
   b) wrapped
   c) placed on abdomen
   d) placed under a special light

8. Vernix caseosa is:
   a) first feeding after 12 hours
   b) an indication of an infection
   c) greasy material that covers the skin of a newborn baby
   d) a sign of fetal distress

9. Lactation:
   a) does not start until the fifth postpartum day
   b) absorbs milk leakage
   c) refers to the flow of milk
   d) is a medicine that suppresses milk production

7.8 Combinations of Verbs and Prepositions

Exercise The meaning of a verb is often determined by the preposition that follows. Example: *to look for* = suchen nach; *to look at* = anschauen.

Complete the following combinations of verbs and prepositions to match the German translations.

1. to call _____ absagen

2. to call _____ kommen um

3. to call _____ vorbeikommen

4. to look _____ sorgen für

5. to look _____ sich umsehen

6. to look _____ aufblicken

7. to send _____ beauftragen, herbeirufen

8. to send _____ verschicken

9. to turn _____ erscheinen

10. to turn _____ schauen

11. to turn _____ ablehnen

12. to turn _____ abschließen

13. to go _____ einschlafen

14. to go _____ fortfahren

15. to go _____ ansteigen

16. to go _____ absinken

17. to bring _____ überzeugen

18. to bring _____ zu Bewusstsein bringen

19. to bring _____ zurückbringen

20. to bring _____ verursachen

7.9 The Obstetrical Patient

Puzzle

Try to fit the following definitions into the puzzle.

1. Helps a baby to get rid of stomach gas.
2. Sound waves with a frequency of over 20,000 Hz which are used to examine the structure of the inside of the body.
3. The portion of the body included in the outlet of the pelvis.
4. A very strong and often painful tightening of a muscle.
5. American word for incubator.
6. A perineal incision made during the birth of a child.
7. Other word for placenta.
8. The state of being a mother.
9. Complication indicated by fever.
10. A small bed for a baby.
11. Stretching or enlargement.
12. Infant during the first four weeks of life.
13. The condition of being pregnant.
14. Other word for 'to nurse', as in 'the mother is nursing her baby'.

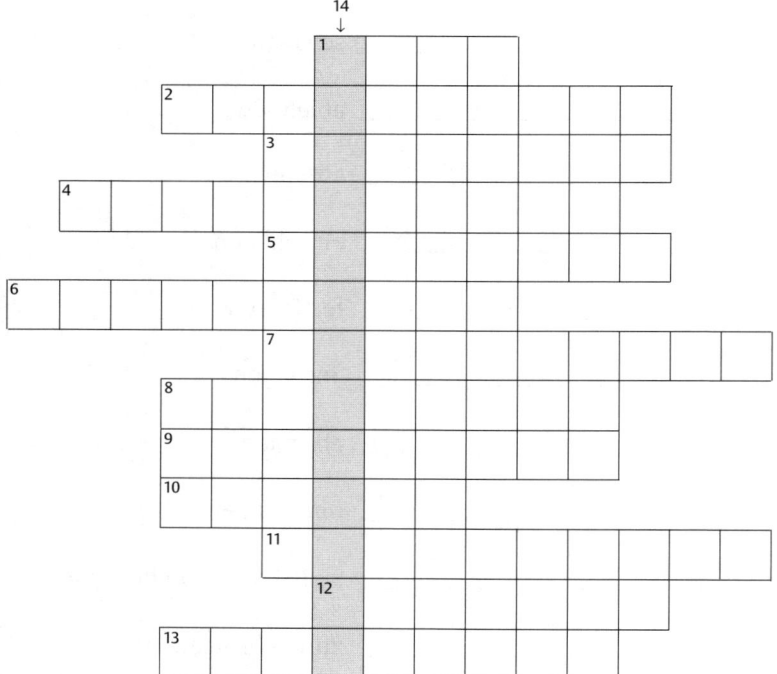

First Aid

8.1 A & E Department

Text

1 Deliberate drug overdose is a common problem in A & E departments. It has been estimated that 110,000 cases of overdose present each year, with 82% of these be-
5 ing admitted and accounting for 14% of all medical admissions.

The majority of patients who attempt suicide (parasuicide) have no intention of killing themselves. In a study of 216 para-
10 suicides, Stanley (1969) found that less than one-quarter had a suicidal intent. Kreitman (1977) describes parasuicide as being carried out at the height of interpersonal crisis, an act which is used as a
15 form of communication and which is designed to give relief from intolerable distress. Studies have shown that alcohol has been taken by 25% of parasuicides.

Paracetamol is one of the drugs used in
20 40% of parasuicides because of the ease with which it can be obtained. However, it is one of the most toxic drugs with as few as 20 tablets (10g) causing hepatotoxicity and possible death; 96% of para-
25 cetamol is metabolised into non-toxic byproduct and excreted unchanged, but 4% is metabolised into a highly toxic substance. Symptoms of hepatotoxicity begin to occur after 24 hours and, after
30 48 hours, jaundice, coagulation defects, hypoglycaemia, renal failure and myocardiopathy may become obvious. Early emergency treatment is indicated.

A stomach wash-out is recommended for
35 overdoses of 20 tablets or more if ingested within 6 hours. Antidotes are effective if given within the 24 hours after ingestion and bind with the toxic metabolite. The stomach wash-out also serves to re-
40 move the alcohol, although this generally would not be indicated if it were the only drug involved. Alcohol causes respiratory depression and in large quantities can cause respiratory arrest.

45 The notion that stomach wash-out teaches the overdose patient a lesson is unsupported. Besides questioning the ethics of such a rationale, there are doubts that parasuicides see the stomach wash-out as
50 a punishment but rather see it in terms of receiving some of the help and attention which they need and desire.

Much care and time must be taken with parasuicides in order to determine their
55 needs and to begin to help them to solve their problems. This is a challenging area to nursing.

Quelle: Adams S. & Tubman G.
Planning patient care: Drug overdose. Melbourne
Macmillan Education ltd.

Try to answer the following questions about the text.

1. *Deliberate* in line 1 means:
   a) to set free
   b) accidental
   c) done on purpose
   d) forced

2. *accounting for* in line 5 means:
   a) to depend on
   b) ask for
   c) to gain
   d) to be the cause of

3. *parasuicide* in line 8 refers to:
   a) an attempted suicide
   b) unintentional suicide
   c) suicide of a paratrooper
   d) a drug overdose

4. *relief* in line 16 means:
   a) ending of anxiety
   b) support
   c) warning
   d) help for people in trouble

5. *obtained* in line 21 means:
   a) stolen
   b) prescribed
   c) to remain in existence
   d) purchased

6. *hepatotoxicity* in line 23/24 refers to:
   a) hepatitis
   b) the injurious effect on liver cells
   c) pancreatitis
   d) poisonous effect on bladder

7. *jaundice* in line 30 means:
   a) shortness of breath
   b) condition in which skin and white part of eyes turn yellow
   c) dizziness
   d) blurred vision

8. *coagulation* in line 30 refers to:
   a) micturition
   b) blood pressure
   c) the process of weakening a liquid
   d) the change from a liquid into a solid state

9. *ingestion* in line 37/38 means:
   a) pain caused by the stomach
   b) stomach wash-out
   c) taking food or medicine into the stomach
   d) defecating

8.2 The Patient at an A & E Department

Conversation

This conversation takes place in the waiting room of an A & E department of a general hospital. The patients' names are *Jack (J), Ruby (R), Ms Daniels (D)* and her daughter *Pam (P),* the nurse's name is *Suzy (S).*

D: *(storming into the room holding a child...)*
   Can somebody please help me! Doctor, nurse, help me please, my child is dying!

S: What is going on here? Okay, calm down, hand me over your child.

D: She's suffocating, nurse, help her quickly, she swallowed one of her marbles, she can't breath, she's all blue!

S: Listen to me, I am going to press my fist into your daughter's abdomen and see if I can push the marble out.
(nurse succeeds after several attempts, the child starts screaming)

P: Mummy, help me, I am going to be sick.

D: Well done nurse, I really thought I was going to lose her. Thank you ever so much.

J: Nurse, what about my hand? I'm bleeding to death!

S: I'll be with you in a minute. You go and sit over there next to the trolley. We will get you stitched up in no time.
(Ruby is brought in on a stretcher)

R: Any chance of getting a drink over here? Hey nurse, come on and give me ...

S: You just be quiet over there, Mr. whatever your name is. According to your breath it will take some time before you are sober again. Maybe we can have a normal conversation then.

J: Nurse, I can't hold this much longer. I think I'm going to faint.

S: There's your doctor coming, he will look after you, so try to relax now.

R: *(singing)* ... and he's a jolly good fellow ...

Translate the following words from the test.

Exercise

1. _____ waiting room

2. _____ suffocating

3. _____ marble

4. _____ abdomen

5. _____ attempts

6. _____ trolley

7. _____ stretcher

8. _____ to stitch up

9. _____ sober

10. _____ to faint

8.3 First Aid

Exercise Are the following statements true or false? *true* *false*

1. A *splinter* is a tiny sliver of wood that gets wedged into the skin. ❏ ❏
2. A *blister* is a mark caused by a blow or fall, resulting in discolouring ❏ ❏
   of the skin.
3. *Tweezers* refers to a small metal tool used for picking up, pulling out ❏ ❏
   and handling very small objects.
4. A *safety pin* is a pin with a guard to cover the point. ❏ ❏
5. A *bruise* is a thin watery swelling under the skin, caused by rubbing ❏ ❏
   or burning.
6. The *Heimlich manoeuvre* is used for people who are drowning. ❏ ❏
7. *Lint* is soft material used for protecting wounds.
8. 'Lint' in the UK is the same as 'fluff' in the USA. ❏ ❏
9. A *dislocation* is the same thing as a fracture. ❏ ❏
10. A *sprained* ankle means that the ligaments which hold the bones to- ❏ ❏
    gether have been overstretched. ❏ ❏

8.4 Emergency phone calls

Dealing with emergency phone calls can be a stressfull business. It is important to speak in a calm and clear voice. Ask for more details when things are not clear.

Exercise

Useful phrases

When did it happen?	Wann ist es geschehen/passiert?
What age is the patient?	Wie alt ist der Patient?
Are there any other known illnesses?	Bestehen andere bekannte (Vor)Erkrankungen?
Is the patient on any medication?	Nimmt der Patient irgendwelche Medikamente?
How long did it take?	Wie lange hat es gedauert?
Is the patient conscious?	Ist der Patient bei Bewusstsein?
Did he/she lose a lot of blood?	Hat er/sie viel Blut verloren?
Has he/she taken any alcohol or drugs?	Hat er/sie Alkohol oder Drogen genommen?
Are there any visible abnormalities?	Zeigen sich sichtbare Abnormalitäten/ Auffälligkeiten?

Below are different situations you can come across. Practice in couples and change roles: one is the patient and one person plays the part of the nurse.

A person phones because:

1. A wound doesn't stop bleeding.
2. Her child doesn't stop vomiting.
3. He found his father unconscious on the floor.
4. Her baby is coming.
5. He has been suffering from diarrhoea for a week.
6. He has taken a double dose of medication by mistake.
7. She has stepped into a glass.
8. He has been bitten by a snake.

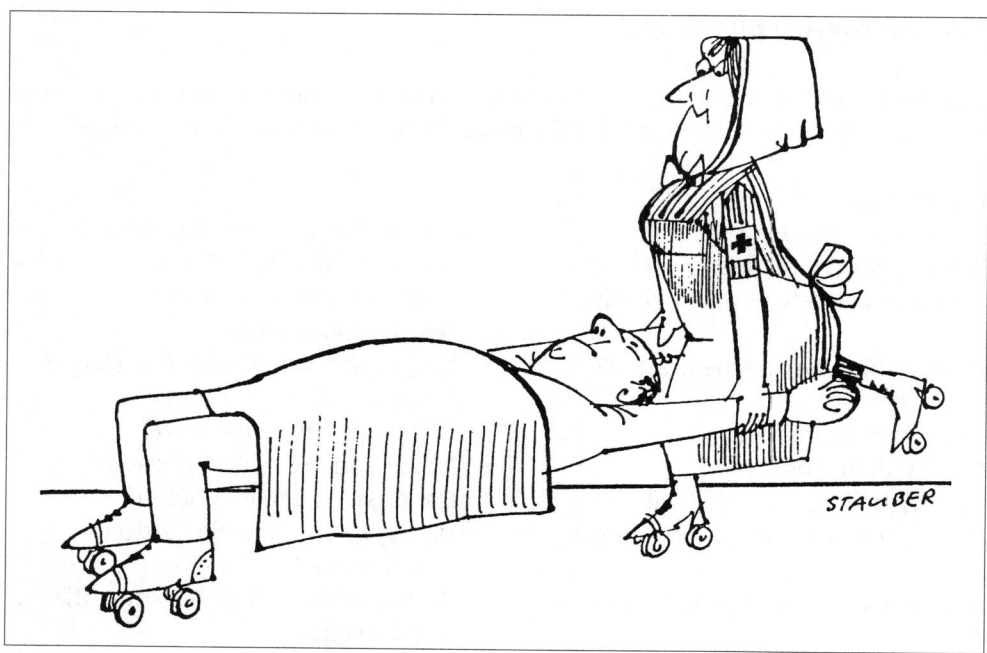

Quelle: Löwensteiner Cartoon Service (Hrsg.): Dr. med. Ironicus. Thieme, Stuttgart 1994 (S. 18)

8.5 The Genitive

Grammar

Um anzugeben, dass etwas jemandem gehört, verwendet man im Englischen „'*s*" oder eine Konstruktion mit „*of*"

1. „'*s*" wird verwendet, wenn es um folgendes geht:

    a) *Personen oder Tiere*

Jane's uniform.	Janes Uniform.
The cat's tail.	Der Schwanz der Katze.

    b) *Zeit, Entfernung oder Gewicht*

This month's rota.	Der Dienstplan dieses Monats.
A mile's walk.	Eine Wanderung von 1,6 km.
An eight-pound's weight.	Ein Gewicht von acht Pfund.

    c) *einen Laden, ein öffentliches Gebäude, Haus etc.*

You can get it at the chemist's.	Es ist beim Drogisten erhältlich.
The party is at Susan's.	Das Fest ist bei Susan.

2. Pluralformen, die mit einem „-s" enden, erhalten ein „'":

A four-months' baby.   Ein Baby von 4 Monaten.

Nurses' tasks.   Aufgaben der Pflegekräfte.

3. Namen, die mit einem „-s" enden, erhalten in der Regel ein „'s":

Mrs Beans's friend.   Der Freund von Frau Beans.

4. Die „*of*"-Konstruktion wird verwendet:

a) *bei Sachen oder Dingen*

The wheels of a trolley.   Die Räder eines kleinen Wagens.

b) *bei Mengen*

A cup of sugar.   Eine Tasse Zucker.

c) *bei geographischen Bezeichnungen*

The port of Dover.   Der Hafen von Dover.

8.6 Translation

Translate the following sentences: *Exercise*

1. Haben Sie bei Ihrer Tante gegessen?

_____

2. Die Arznei des Mädchens.

_____

3. Soll ich Ihnen eine Tasse Tee bringen?

_____

4. Er arbeitet beim Fleischer.

_____

5. Es gibt eine Anzahl von Dingen.

_____

8.7 Reasons for Older People to Attend an A & E Department

1 A study was conducted to identify any shortfalls in the discharge of older people from A & E departments and areas in which improvements could be made. The 5 conclusions that could be drawn were:
– a large percentage of older people attending A & E departments may have conditions which could be easily treated by their general practitioners;
10 – many of the older people whose attendances might be classified as 'inappropriate' live alone.

Health visitors could play an important part in ensuring that older people receive 15 appropriate treatment, reducing the load on already stretched A & E departments:
– checklists could be useful in ensuring that older people are discharged from A & E departments with an assurance of 20 adequate follow-up.
– further research into 'unjustifiable' attendances is essential.

Quelle: *Nursing Times* 1995; 91 (13).

Exercise

Translate the following words from the text.

1. _____ Behandlung

2. _____ unangebracht

3. _____ Belastung

4. _____ klassifiziert

5. _____ nicht zu verantworten

6. _____ Mängel

7. _____ ausreichend

8. _____ viel Betrieb

8.8 Resuscitation

Information

Airway

The maintenance of the casualty's airway is a priority. If breathing has stopped, artificial ventilation must be started immediately. If the lungs do not receive air, the brain will be deprived of oxygen, which will quickly result in unconsciousness and cardiac arrest.

Obstruction

There is a danger that the tongue could block the air passage, so the head and jaw should always be drawn forward. Choking is largely caused by spasm, but may also be caused by the presence of a foreign body. If there is an obvious obstruction, remove it. To dislodge an obstruction from a child's windpipe, you should sit in a chair or on one knee and lay the child over your knee, head down and apply a few sharp slaps between the shoulders. Three or four sharp slaps between an adult's shoulders may also clear the airway, especially if the casualty bends over so that the head is lower than the lungs.

Breathing

Mouth-to-mouth ventilation
This method provides the greatest ventilation of the lungs and oxygenation of the blood. During application, the movement of the chest can be observed to assess how the lungs are inflating. Method:
- lay casualty on his or her back
- with one hand on top of the casualty's head and the other supporting the neck, tilt the head back
- transfer your hand from the neck and push the casualty's chin upwards
- lift the jaw upwards and forwards to prevent the tongue from blocking the airway
- open the casualty's mouth and pinch the casualty's nostrils together with your thumb and forefinger
- take a deep breath in, then place your mouth over the casualty's mouth, and exhale into the casualty's lungs
- observe movement of the casualty's chest, to ensure that it rises
- remove your mouth and watch the chest deflate.

Repeat this procedure, giving the first four breaths as quickly as possible.

Cardiac Massage

Do not continue ventilation alone if the casualty's heart is not beating, as the oxygenated blood will not be able to circulate. To make certain that the heart has stopped beating, check the patient's pulse in the carotid artery at the neck. If there is a very faint heartbeat, do not attempt external cardiac compression. However, if the heart has stopped, carry out the following steps:

- place the casualty on a firm surface on his/her back
- kneel at the casualty's side
- place the heel of one hand on the lower half of the sternum
- place the heel of the other hand over the already positioned hand and lock the fingers together
- keeping the arms straight, rock forwards and press down on the lower half of the sternum
- rock backwards to release pressure
- repeat movement once per second
- continue ventilation with 5 cardiac compressions to each ventilation.

If resuscitation is successful, the carotid pulse will return and the colour of the casualty's face will improve. As soon as the heartbeat returns, stop applying the compressions.

Quelle: *First aid. Nurses' Dictionary*. Edinburgh: Churchill Livingstone.

Exercise

Translate the following words from the text.

1. _____ maintenance

2. _____ artificial ventilation

3. _____ deprived of

4. _____ unconsciousness

5. _____ cardiac arrest

6. _____ block

7. _____ air passage

8. _____ jaw

9. _____ choking

10. _____ dislodge

11. _____ windpipe

12. _____ slaps

13. _____ oxygenation

14. _____ inflating

15. _____ tilt

16. _____ nostrils

17. _____ pinch

18. _____ carotid artery

19. _____ faint

20. _____ rock

8.9 Different Meanings

Exercise

Depending on the context words can have different meanings, for example: *a drug* refers to (a) a medicine or (b) a substance one takes as a habit for leasure or excitement.

Try to complete the missing meaning.

1. *a pint*   **a)** a drink of beer

   b) _____

2. *a sister*   **a)** female sibling

   b) _____

3. *father*   **a)** a male parent

   b) _____

4. *to pinch*   **a)** to press between thumb and finger

   b) _____

5. *to arrest*   **a)** to seize by the power of the law

   b) _____

6. *to nurse*   **a)** to look after a patient

            b) _____

7. *sweat*   **a)** perspiration

            b) _____

8. *a cap*   **a)** diaphragm (also 'Dutch cap')

            b) _____

9. *a cable*   **a)** a thick strong metal rope

            b) _____

10. *thick*   **a)** having a large distance between opposite surfaces

            b) _____

Measures and Abbreviations

9.1 Mission Impossible

1 So, there I was, my first working day in the UK. It had taken ages before the UKCC registered me as an RGN, but finally everything was OK. I had to start at 7 am on a
5 Care of the Elderly ward. I was looking forward to work again. The only problem was that nobody had told me I would now be entering the 'abbreviation zone'! It started with the handover by the CN.
10 'Mr Johnson, known with a COAD and CHF, is leaving today AMA. His wife does insist on his discharge. For Mr Cleveland, who was admitted yesterday with LVF, we still need an ASU. Mr Roslin's NG can be re-
15 moved today, since he is eating much better. Mrs Davies, admitted with a PE, can have her medication PRN. Her family decided for a DNR. Miss Waley, recovering from a BKA, needs assistance with her ex-
20 ercises TID. Mrs Lurch, known with SDAT and severe NVD, was less confused last night, she will continue her TPN as tol.' While the sister continued her report I stopped writing. There was no way I was
25 going to understand what she was saying, so I just hoped for the best when we were finally dismissed. My colleagues ordered me around to help patients OOB a.s.a.p. Af-ter they were all washed and dressed I
30 started doing the q2h CKS.
Let me take somebody's BP any time, that is easy enough. But although I could work out what BP & T meant, I was puzzled by the abbreviations BM & PU. I knew what
35 BM could mean in German but I did not think it referred to the same thing here and PU I had never heard of. I was racking my brains for combinations like potassium something..., but that did not make
40 any sense either.
Besides, these letters were on every PT's chart, so surely it had to be something simple. The solution came when a nurse told me to bring an ASU and a faeces spec-
45 imen from Mr Roslin to the lab. 'By the way', she said, 'you can also put a cross and your initials on his BM & PU list.' 'What do you mean?' I asked, not knowing what was going on and probably look-
50 ing very sheepishly. 'Well, it is obvious he moved his bowels and passed urine, is it not,' she answered while pointing at the samples I was holding in my hand. By that time I thought working here would be an
5 MI, or mission impossible ...

Try to find the right explanation for the following abbreviations from the text, using the descriptions on the next page.

1. _____ UK

2. _____ UKCC

3. _____ RGN

4. _____ OK

5. _____ am

6. _____ CN

7. _____ COAD

8. _____ CHF

9. _____ AMA

10. _____ LVF

11. _____ ASU

12. _____ NG

13. _____ PE

14. _____ PRN

15. _____ DNR

16. _____ BKA

17. _____ TID

18. _____ SDAT

19. _____ NVD

20. _____ TPN

21. _____ as tol.

22. _____ OOB

23. _____ a.s.a.p.

24. _____ q2h

25. _____ CKS

26. _____ BP & T

27. _____ PTS

28. _____ lab.

29. _____ BM

30. _____ PU

out of bed   below-knee amputation   patient's   laboratory   passed urine   ante meridiem   (Latin; 'before noon')   checks   chronic heart failure   senile dementia of Alzheimer's type   blood pressure and temperature   United Kingdom   charge nurse bowel movement   as tolerated   total parenteral nutrition   every two hours (Latin: quaque 2 hora) United Kingdom Central Council (for Nursing, Midwifery and Health Visiting)   as soon as possible   per requestum   Registered General Nurse   all correct against medical advice   nausea, vomiting, diarrhoea   do not resuscitate   nasogastric tube   chronic obstructive airway disease   three times a day (Latin: ter in die)   pulmonary embolism   left ventricle failure   admission specimen urine

9.2 Translation

Note on abbreviations and acronyms: In modern usage Latin expressions are alternately used as an abbreviation or as an acronym. Abbreviations are shortened forms of words, often using lower-case letters and full stops: t.i.d. = ter in die. Unlike abbreviations, acronyms are pronounced as words rather than as just a series of letters. They are mostly written in capital letters, as in TID.

Fill in the German translation of the following abbreviations.   _Exercise_

1. _____ DOB   date of birth

2. _____ UK   unknown

3. _____ R/O   ruled out

4. _____ ht   height

5.	_____	wt	weight
6.	_____	Rx	treatment
7.	_____	Fx	fracture
8.	_____	abd	abdomen
9.	_____	jt	joint
10.	_____	LBP	low back pain
11.	_____	ad lib	as desired
12.	_____	cl liq	clear liquid
13.	_____	stat	at once
14.	_____	top	topically
15.	_____	amb	ambulatory
16.	_____	MH	marital history
17.	_____	alt noct	alternate nights
18.	_____	q.s.	sufficient quantity
19.	_____	OPD	outpatient department
20.	_____	SIDS	sudden infant death syndrome

9.3 Diplomas and Degrees in the Health Service

Information

Bachelor:	4jährige HBO-Ausbildung
Diploma:	ca. 3jährige HBO/Inservice-Ausbildung
Doctor/PhD:	Doktortitel nach abgeschlossener Dissertation
Master:	4jährige Universitätsausbildung

ADNS	Assistant Director of Nursing Services
AN	Ancillary Nurse (auch: NA)
BASC	Bachelor of Applied Science
BEd	Bachelor of Education
BHyg	Bachelor of Hygiene
BM	Bachelor of Medicine (auch: MB)
BN	Bachelor of Nursing (auch: *BSN*, S=Science)
BPharm	Bachelor of Pharmacy
BSC	Bachelor of Science
CMT	Clinical Midwife Teacher
CNN	Certificated Nursery Nurse
CNO	Chief Nursing Officer
CNT	Clinical Nurse Teacher
Dch	Doctor of Surgery
DCH	Diploma in Child Health
DchD	Doctor of Dental Surgery
DCM	Diploma in Community Medicine
DCMT	Diploma in Clinical Medicine of Tropics
DEN	District Enrolled Nurse
DipN	Diploma in Nursing (auch: *DN*)
DM	Doctor of Medicine (auch: *MD*)
DMHS	Director of Medical and Health Services
DMT	District Management Team
DN	District Nurse
DNE	Diploma in Nursing Education
DNS	Director of Nursing Services
EN(G)	Enrolled Nurse (General)
EN(M)	Enrolled Nurse (Mental)
EN(MH)	Enrolled Nurse (Mental Handicap)
FETC	Further Education Teaching Certificate
FRCn	Fellow of the Royal College of Nursing
GP	General Practitioner
HV	Health Visitor
LM	Licentiate in Midwifery
LPN	Licensed Practical Nurse (auch: *LVN*)
LVN	Licensed Vocational Nurse (auch: *LPN*)
MA	Master of Arts
MAO	Master of the Art of Obstetrics (auch: *MO*)
MEd	Master of Education
MPH	Master of Public Health
MSC	Master of Science
MSOCSC	Master of Social Science (auch: *MSciscoc*)

MO	Medical Officer
MSW	Medical Social Worker
NA	Nursing Assistant (auch: *AN*)
ODA	Operating Department Assistant
OHNC	Occupational Health Nurse Certificate
OT	Occupational Therapist
PhD	doctoral degree (auch: *Doctor of Philosophy*)
PT	Physiotherapist
RCNT	Registered Clinical Nurse Teacher
RGN	Registered General Nurse
RM	Registered Midwife
RMN	Registered Mental Nurse
RN	Registered Nurse (auch: *SRN*; S=State)
RNMH	Registered Nurse for the Mentally Handicapped
RSCN	Registered Sick Children Nurse
SHO	Senior House Officer

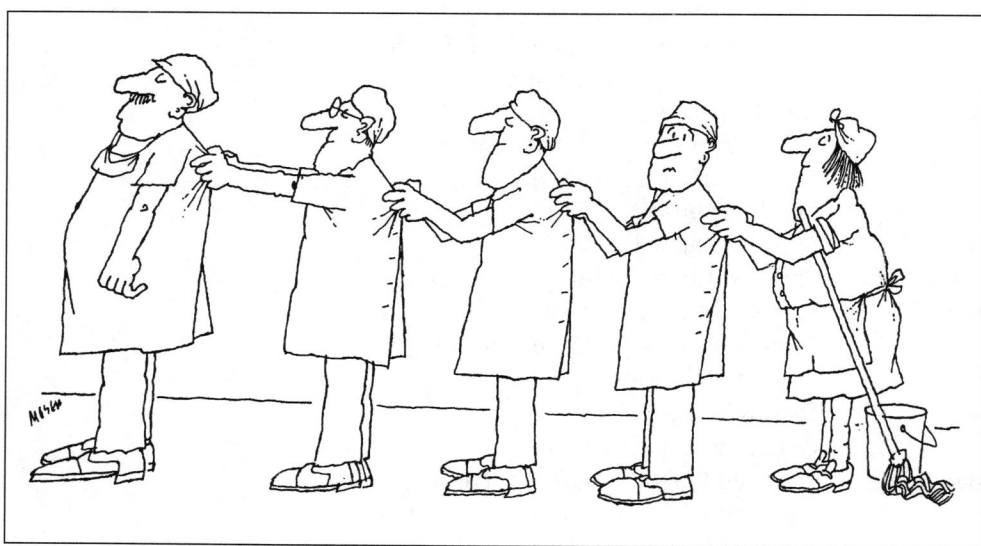

Quelle: Löwensteiner Cartoon Service (Hrsg.): Dr. med. Ironicus. Thieme, Stuttgart 1994 (S. 73)

9.4 Nursing Education in the USA

Text

Nursing education evolved from the model developed by Florence Nightingale based on her experiences in military hospitals during the Crimean War (1853-1856). Hospital-based and heavily work-orientated this apprenticeship model dominated education of nurses until the years following the Second World War, when the shift towards colleges and universities gained momentum. The Goldmark report in 1923 began a continuing debate about the appropriate entry level for nursing, with consensus forming around two levels: professional and associate, both requiring college or university preparation.

Nursing education has matured considerably in the US since its beginning in 1873. The curriculum has been enlarged to accommodate increased scientific and health knowledge. Students are more thoroughly grounded in theory, psychosocial aspects are emphasized, as is the wellness model, and services to patients are no longer provided by students. Clinical experiences have become truly educational experiences. Postgraduate education has a high priority, with many nurses enrolled in programmes leading to master's and doctoral degrees. The two categories of basic education for licensed nurses are registered nurses (RNS) and practical nurses (LPNS).

Currently, education for licensure as a registered nurse is offered in three types of programmes, all requiring high-school certificates for entry.

Newest of the three programmes, initiated in 1952, the associate programme is usually located in a two-year community college course and confers an associate degree (AD). Oldest of the three programmes, diploma study is located in hospitals. A diploma is offered after three years' training. Academic courses are usually provided by educational institutions or two-year or four-year college courses. The four-year baccalaureate programme in colleges and universities leads to a bachelor's degree in nursing.

The usual pattern is a two-year nursing major after two years of course work in the sciences and liberal arts. In addition there are a few programmes that offer master's or doctoral degrees as basic education for entry into practice. However, these are extremely rare and will probably not become more numerous in the future.

Quelle: Levine e.a. *Nursing Practice in the UK and North America*. London: Chapman & Hall.

Translate the following words from the text.

Exercise

1. apprenticeship (l. 6)	...	**a)** Hauptfach
2. shift (l. 9)	...	**b)** entwickelt
3. momentum (l. 10)	...	**c)** Registrierung
4. entry level (l. 12)	...	**d)** Lehre
5. matured (l. 16)	...	**e)** zahlreich
6. grounded (l. 22)	...	**f)** Verschiebung

7. postgraduate (l. 27/28)	… **g)**	führt zu
8. enrolled (l. 29)	… **h)**	Stoßkraft
9. licensure (l. 34)	… **i)**	postdoktoral
10. confers (l. 41)	… **j)**	Zulassungsanforderung
11. major (l. 52)	… **k)**	Alphafächer
12. liberal arts (l. 53)	… **l)**	gute Vorbildung
13. numerous (l. 58)	… **m)**	eingeschrieben

9.5 Comparisons (Steigerungsstufen)

Grammar

Im Englischen unterscheidet man zwischen dem Komparativ und dem Superlativ. Diese werden gebildet:

1. indem man an das Adjektiv, das in der Aussprache *einsilbig* ist, „*-er*" oder „*-est*" anhängt:

short	short**er**	short**est**
weak	weak**er**	weak**est**

ebenso an *zweisilbige* Adjektive, die auf „*-er, -le, -ow, -y, -some*" enden:

happy	happi**er**	happi**est**
lonesome	lonesom**er**	lonesom**est**

und an *zweisilbige* Adjektive mit *Betonung* auf der *2. Silbe*:

polite	polit**er**	polit**est**
severe	sever**er**	sever**est**

2. *zweisilbige* Adjektive, die nicht unter **1.** fallen, und Adjektive, die *länger* sind *als zwei Silben*, erhalten als Hinzufügung „*more*" oder „*most*"

wonderful	**more** wonderful	**most** wonderful
comfortable	**more** comfortable	**most** comfortable

3. *unregelmäßige* Steigerungsstufen:

good	better	best
bad	worse	worst
little	less	least
much/many	more	most

Exercise

Fill in the correct form.

1. It was _____ than we thought. (schlechter)

2. Ron and Harry are the _____ researchers I have ever known. (fröhlichsten)

3. This is the _____ position for you. (bequemster)

4. The girl became _____ every day. (dünner)

5. Danielle did not overlook the _____ detail. (kleinster)

6. We will have to find a _____ tube. (kleiner)

7. He is behaving _____ every day. (unvorsichtiger)

8. That uniform is even _____ than Wilma's. (dreckiger)

9. The _____ ward of the hospital. (stressigster)

10. That operation was the _____ event of the year. (spannendster)

9.6 Measurements

In englischsprachigen Ländern benutzt man verschiedene Abmessungen, Hohlmaße und Gewichtsbestimmungen, die in Deutschland nicht verwendet werden. Hier folgt eine Übersicht: *Information*

Metric System

linear measure: Längenmaß

			1 millimetre	=	0.039	inch (in)
10	mm	=	1 centimetre	=	0.394	in
10	cm	=	1 decimetre	=	3.94	in
10	dm	=	1 metre	=	39.37	in
1000	m	=	1 kilometre	=	0.6214	mile

square measure: Flächenmaß

			1 sq centimetre	=	0.155	sq in
10,000	cm^2	=	1 sq metre	=	1.196	sq yd
100	m^2	=	1 are	=	119.6	sq yd
100	ares	=	1 hectare	=	2.471	acres
100	ha	=	1 sq kilometre	=	0.386	sq miles

cubic measure: Hohlmaß

		1 cu centimetre	=	0.061	in^3
1000 cu cm	=	1 cu decimetre	=	0.035	ft^3
1000 cu dm	=	1 cu metre	=	1.308	yd^3

capacity measure: Hohlmaß (Volumen)

			1 millilitre	=	0.002	pint (pt)
10	ml	=	1 centilitre	=	0.018	pt
10	cl	=	1 decilitre	=	0.176	pt
10	dl	=	1 litre	=	1.76	pt
1000	l	=	1 kilolitre	=	220.0	gallon (gall)

weight: Gewicht

			1 milligram	=	0.015	grain (gr)
10	mg	=	1 centigram	=	0.154	grain
10	cg	=	1 decigram	=	1.543	grain
10	dg	=	1 gram (gr)	=	15.43	grain
					0.035	ounce (oz)
1000	g	=	1 kilogram	=	2.205	pound (lb)
1000	kg	=	1 tonne	=	0.984	(long) ton

Imperial System (britisches System)

linear measure

1 inch	=	25.4	mm
1 foot	=	0.305	mm
1 yard	=	0.914	m
1 mile	=	1.61	km

capacity measure

1 fluid ounce	=	28.4	cm^3
1 pint	=	0.568	dm^3
1 quart	=	1.136	dm^3
1 gallon	=	4.546	dm^3

weight

1 grain	=	64.8	mg
1 dram	=	1.772	g
1 ounce	=	28.35	g
1 pound	=	0.4536	kg
1 stone	=	6.35	kg
1 quarter	=	12.7	kg
1 ton	=	1.016	tonnes
1 short ton	=	0.907	tonnes

9.7 Problem Statements in Patient Reports

Assessment of the patient's health status is an ongoing activity. Clarity and conciseness will help to ensure communication among the health carers. Try to translate the following terms that may be useful in stating patient problems.

Exercise

1. _____ insufficient

2. _____ increase

3. _____ unable to

4. _____ alteration in

5. _____ mood swing

6. _____ impairment of

7. _____ inappropriate

8. _____ reduced

9. _____ mögliche Gefahr

10. _____ Fortschritt

11. _____ entgegenarbeiten

12. _____ eingeschränkt

13. _____ Unvermögen

14. _____ Probleme mit

15. _____ Verlust an

9.8 Translation

Exercise   Translate the following sentences.

1. Verschlechterte Mobilität durch Krampfadern.

---

2. Beschränkte Bewegungsabläufe in den Gelenken durch Gelenkentzündung.

---

3. Fühlt sich depressiv und kann nicht länger in diesem Zustand bleiben.

---

4. Äußert Sorgen bezüglich der Einschaltung des Sozialdienstes.

---

5. Kann das Bett nicht verlassen oder selbständig laufen.

---

6. Angst vor dem Verlassenwerden durch Krankenhausaufnahme.

---

7. Mögliche Infektion durch verringerte Widerstandskräfte.

---

8. Neigung zum Hinfallen.

---

9. Patient will sich nicht äußern.

---

10. Es sollte besprochen werden, wie das Problem vom Patienten selbst gesehen wird.

9.9 Abbreviations

Match the following abbreviations with the explanations on the next page. *Exercise*

time abbreviations

1. _____ AC

2. _____ alt dieb

3. _____ alt hor

4. _____ BID

5. _____ BIN

6. _____ h

7. _____ HS

8. _____ noc(t)

9. _____ pm

10. _____ QD

11. _____ QH

12. _____ QID

13. _____ QM

14. _____ QN

15. _____ QOD

patient charting

16. _____ ADT

17. _____ BR

18. _____ BRP

19. _____ DC

20. _____ DNI

21. _____ Dx

22. _____ Hx

23. _____ NA

24. _____ N/C

25. _____ NPO

26. _____ Px

27. _____ Sx

28. _____ YOB

four times a day   not applicable   before meals   symptoms   bathroom privileges   hour every other day   prognosis   twice a night   year of birth   every morning   night   alternate days/every other day   discontinue   admission, discharge, transfer   alternate hours   twice a day   post meridiem/after noon   bed rest   nothing by mouth   no complaints   hour of sleep   every day   history   every hour   do not intubate   every night diagnosis

Anatomy

10.1 The respiratory system

Text

1 The respiratory system is one of the most vital systems in the human body. In health, it functions automatically and usually without awareness. There are, 5 however, few disease processes that do not have some disruptive effect on the respiratory system. There are also many respiratory disorders relating to environmental pollution, trauma, infection, ge- 10 netic susceptibility and primary disease, as well as conditions secondary to other diseases. Although causative agents differ, the aetiology of each condition follows certain common patterns. To know 15 the anatomy and physiology of the respiratory system is to understand how respiratory disorders inevitably relate to breakdown in ventilation, gaseous exchange or pulmonary perfusion. Symp- 20 toms differ only in degree and effect, and the treatment of symptoms will always have certain basic aims.

The effects of respiratory disorders range from the minor discomforts of the com- 25 mon cold to the distressing and life- threatening symptoms associated with respiratory failure. All are disabling to some extent to the individual and his family. As respiratory conditions and 30 diseases cover such a broad spectrum and are common in both community and hospital settings, it is essential that nurses have a broad knowledge base relating to the basic concepts of normal respiration 35 and an understanding of the factors that can lead to respiratory dysfunction.

Research indicates that some of the more serious respiratory disorders are related to lifestyle and are actually preventable. 40 Nursing care should therefore emphasize on health promotion and disease prevention and the nurse's expanding role, opportunities and challenges in this field. Nurses should, however, work in close 45 collaboration with other health care professionals and, in many instances, are responsible for coordinating the work of the whole team.

Quelle: Alexander e.a. *Nursing Practice Hospital & Home, The Adult.* Churchill Livingstone, 2000.

Exercise   Try to answer the following questions about the text.

1. awareness in line 4 refers to:
   a) any harm
   b) effort
   c) strain
   d) having knowledge

2. disruptive in line 6 means:
   a) to bring into disorder
   b) positive
   c) great
   d) benefical

3. susceptibility in line 10 means:
   a) preference
   b) likelihood to suffer from
   c) engineering
   d) disease

4. agents in line 12 means:
   a) spies
   b) medicines
   c) laws
   d) a thing that produces an effect

5. inevitably in line 17 means:
   a) which cannot be avoided
   b) always
   c) sometimes
   d) which cannot be heard

6. cold in line 25 refers to:
   a) absence of heat
   b) flu
   c) lack of feeling
   d) an illness esp. of the nose and throat

7. disabling in line 27 means:
   a) disconnecting
   b) separating
   c) make unable to use body properly
   d) disheartening

8. to emphasize in line 40 means:
   a) to force
   b) to question
   c) to pay special attention
   d) to stimulate

9. collaboration in line 45 means:
   a) control
   b) cooperation
   c) opposition
   d) examination

10.2 The Human Body and Hand

Fill in the right names for the different parts of the body and hand.

body

1. _____

2. _____

3. _____

4. _____

5. _____

6. _____

7. _____

8. _____

9. _____

10. _____

11. _____

12. _____

hand

13. _____

14. _____

15. _____

16. _____

17. _____

18. _____

10.3 The Human Body and Foot

Exercise   Fill in the right names for the different parts of the body and foot.

body

1. _____

2. _____

3. _____

4. _____

5. _____

6. _____

7. _____

8. _____

9. _____

10. _____

11. _____

12. _____

foot

13. _____

14. _____

15. _____

16. _____

17. _____

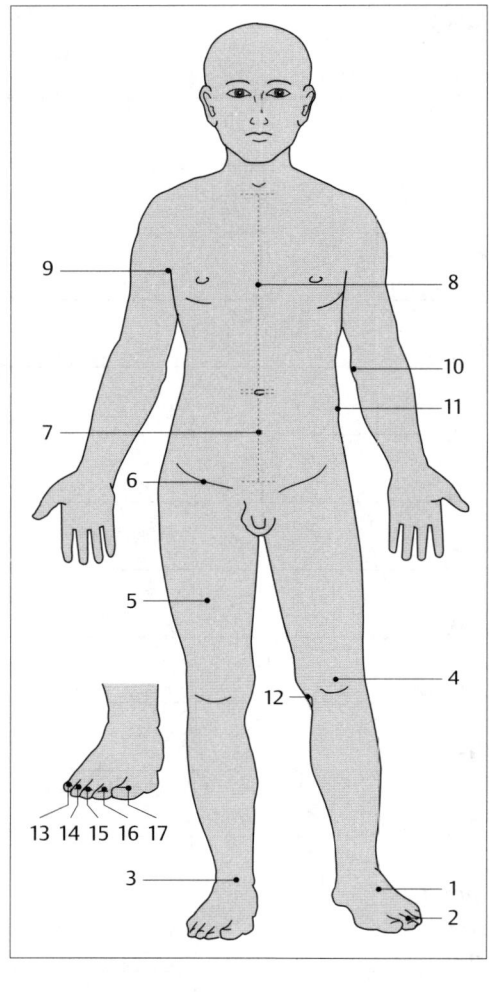

10.4 Adjectives and Adverbs

Grammar

Adjectives are words that describe nouns or pronouns
>The news was *bad.*
>She is a *careful* person.

Adjektive werden auch nach Verben sinnlicher Wahrnehmung verwendet.
>I'm feeling *fine.*
>The food smells *good.*

Adverbs are words or groups of words that describe or add to the meaning of a verb, an adjective, another adverb or a whole sentence.
>They *carefully* handed over the child.
>The news was *very* bad.
>It happened *surprisingly* quickly.
>*Naturally,* she will see you today.

Ein Adverb wird meistens durch das **Adjektiv + „-ly"** gebildet.
>real   **really**
>bad   **badly**

Ausnahmen:
Das Adverb von *good* ist **well.**
>She is a *good* surgeon.   She operates *well.*

Einige Adverbien haben die gleiche Form wie das Adjektiv.
>The drugs were *cheap.*   They bought them *cheap.*
>He was *pretty.*   That was *pretty* mean.
>I was on an *early* shift.   They arrived *early.*
>It is *hard* to know.   She tried very *hard.*

Exercise

Fill in the right adjective or adverb.

1. He is a _____ smoker. (stark)

2. The limb had _____ recovered. (vollständig)

3. His head was _____ damaged. (ernsthaft)

4. Necrosis often demands _____ operation. (frühzeitig)

5. The back of his arm was _____ bruised. (stark)

6. A small fracture is_____ overlooked. (einfach)

7. I _____ know him. (kaum)

8. The spine consists of 24 separate _____ shaped bones. (verschieden)

9. The skeleton is _____ flexible. (merklich)

10. Injury to the soft tissue is often _____. (groß)

10.5 Translation

Exercise

Translate the following sentences.

1. Die einzige Behandlung, die nötig ist, besteht aus Ruhigstellung durch einen Gipsverband.

   _____

2. Die sinnlichen Eigenschaften von Geschmacks- und Geruchssinn sind eng miteinander verbunden.

   _____

3. Zerkaute Nahrung geht erst durch die Speiseröhre.

   _____

4. Das Herz des Kindes schlägt unregelmäßig.

   _____

5. Er kann kaum stehen.

   _____

10.6 Body Organs

Exercise

Fill in the gaps, using the words below.

stomach   rectum   larynx   kidneys   colon   duodenum [d(j)u:əʊ'di:nəm]   *trachea* ['treɪki:ə]   *bladder   spleen   diaphragm   thyroid*

The trunk of the body contains two large cavities separated by a muscular sheet called the (1) _____. The most dilated part of the digestive tube, situated between the oesophagus and the beginning of the small intestine, is the (2) _____, which plays a role in digesting food. At the tail of the pancreas, behind the stomach, the (3) _____ is situated. It controls the quality of the blood supply and produces certain blood cells. The urinary system consists of the (4) _____ which are responsible for the excretion of nitrogenous wastes and the (5) _____. The first of the three parts of the small intestine is called the (6) _____, which extends from the pylorus of the stomach to the jejunum. The (7) _____ is the main part of the large intestine, which consists of four sections. It absorbs large amounts of water and electrolytes from the undigested food passed on from the small intestine. At intervals peristaltic movements transport the contents towards the (8) _____. At the upper end of the throat lies a boxlike part in which the sounds of the voice are produced. This organ is called the (9) _____. The (10) _____ gland is found on both sides of the (11) _____. It secretes thyroxine, which controls the rate of metabolism.

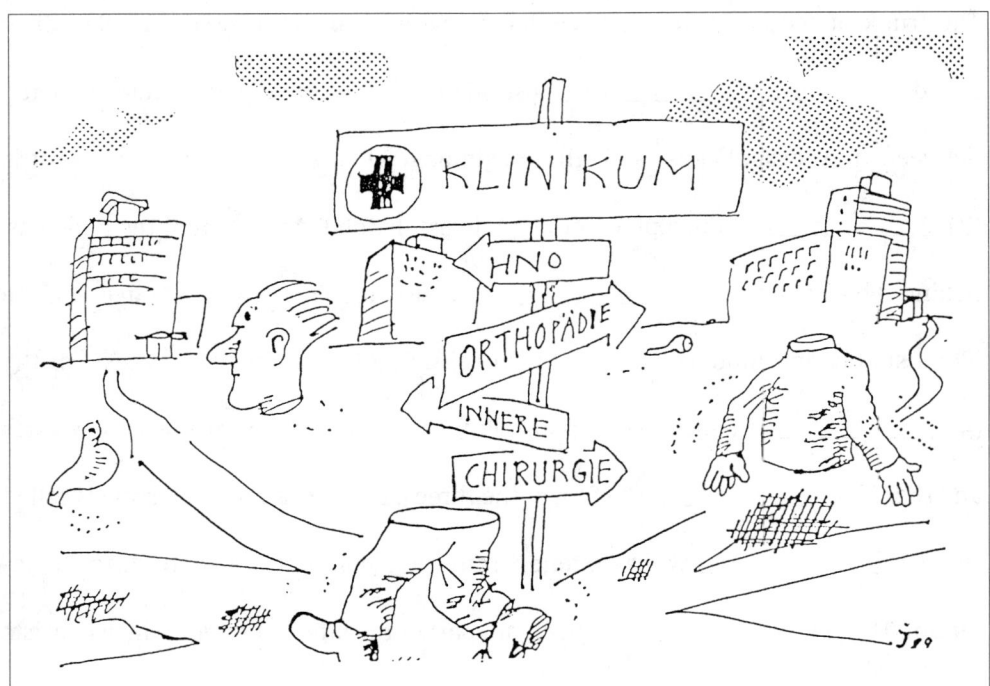

Quelle: Löwensteiner Cartoon Service (Hrsg.): Dr. med. Ironicus. Thieme, Stuttgart 1994 (S. 66)

10.7 Frequently-Used Verbs

Exercise   Translate the following verbs.

1. _____ verbessern

2. _____ ermutigen

3. _____ sterilisieren

4. _____ desinfizieren

5. _____ bewerten

6. _____ beurteilen

7. _____ assistieren

8. _____ koordinieren

9. _____ abstimmen

10. _____ abschließen

11. _____ unterbrechen

12. _____ verfolgen

13. _____ hinterfragen

14. _____ untersuchen

15. _____ reanimieren

16. _____ unterstützen

17. _____ einspritzen

18. _____ aufgeben

19. _____ einstellen

20. _____ einbringen

21. _____ bewältigen

22. _____ benötigen

23. _____ ausdrücken

24. _____ besprechen

25. _____ lindern/mildern

26. _____ regeln

27. _____ führen zu

28. _____ einschätzen

29. _____ verursachen

30. _____ hinweisen auf

10.8 Bones of the Skeleton

Exercise

Fill in the right names for the different parts of the skeleton, using the words on the next page.

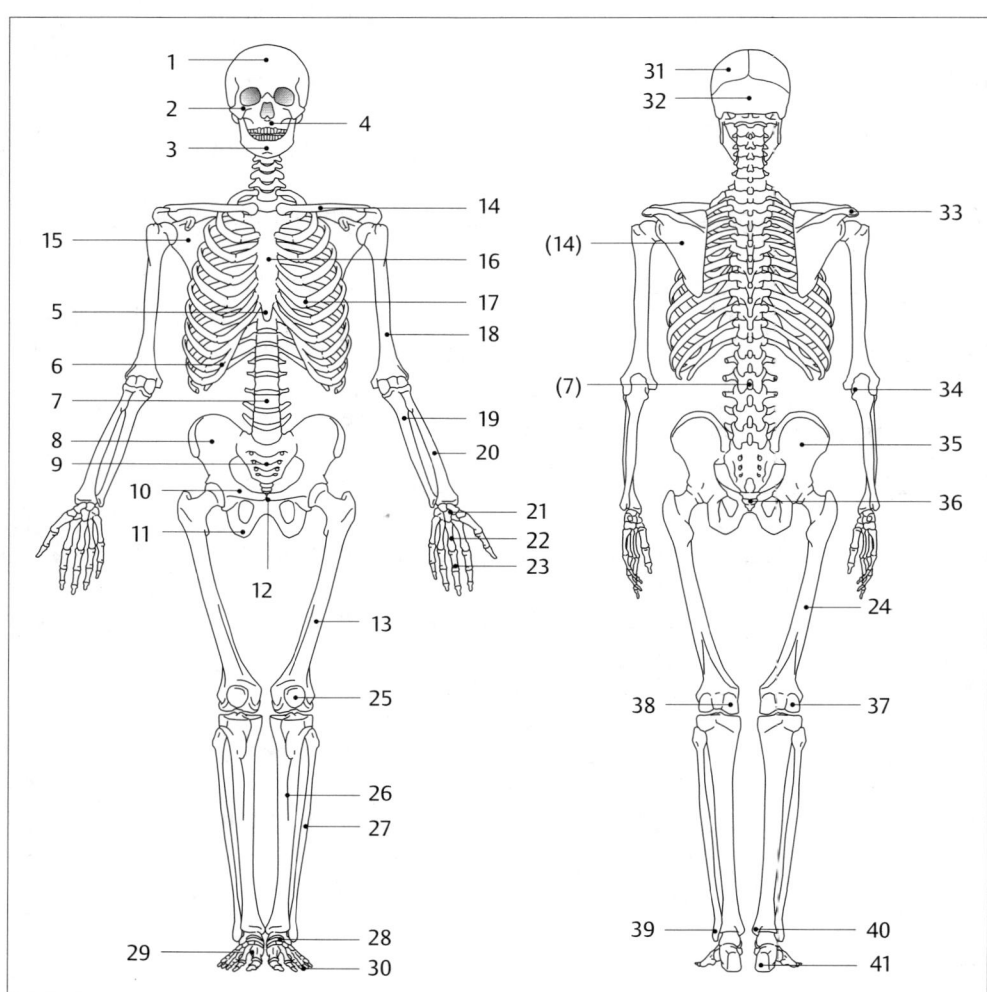

skull
1. _____
2. _____
3. _____
4. _____
31. _____
32. _____

thorax
5. _____
6. _____
7. _____
16. _____
17. _____

pelvic girdle
8. _____
9. _____
10. _____
11. _____
12. _____
36. _____

shoulder girdle
14. _____
15. _____
33. _____

upper extremity
18. _____
19. _____
20. _____
21. _____
22. _____
23. _____
34. _____

lower extremity
13. _____
24. _____
25. _____
26. _____
27. _____
28. _____
29. _____
30. _____
37. _____
38. _____
39. _____
40. _____
41. _____

parietal
femur
femur
clavicle
cranium

symphysis pubis
  ['sɪmfəsɪs]
lateral condyle ['kandaɪl]
medial condyle
xiphoid ['zɪfɔɪd] process
mandible ['mændɪbl]
calcaneus [kæl'keɪnɪəs]
carpals ['kɑːrpəls]
ulna
patella
zygomatic bone
metacarpals
phalanges
phalanges [fə'lænʤɪːz]
humerus
olecranon [əʊ'lekrənɑn]
scapula
maxilla
ilium
lateral malleolus/maleo-
  lus (USA) [mə'lɪələs]/
  outer ankle
medial malleolus/inner
  ankle
pubis
costal cartilage
ribs
coccyx ['kaksɪks]
occipital bone [ak'sɪpɪtl]
acromion
vertebral column
pelvic girdle
metatarsals
tarsal
fibula ['fɪbjələ]
tibia
radius
sternum
sacrum
ischium ['ɪskɪəm]

10.9 The Human Body

Puzzle Try to fit the translations of the following words into the puzzle.

1. Wadenbein
2. Gelenk
3. Pankreas
4. Vorhaut
5. Gebärmutter
6. Schilddrüse
7. Bronchien
8. Mandeln
9. Gelenkband
10. Milz
11. Prostata
12. Bauchfell
13. Zunge
14. Harnleiter
15. Well done! This is your …

Nursing Process

11.1 Comparing Qualified Nurse and Auxiliary Roles

Text

An occasional paper in *Nursing times* describes the contribution of nursing auxiliaries (NAs) compared with qualified nurses (QNs) in terms of activities performed. It also examines how this was affected by three organisational types, namely primary, team and functional nursing. Twelve QNs and 12 NAs were chosen randomly in each organisational type. Data were collected using non participant observation and a computerised event recorder. The most interesting findings were found *across* organizational type, with QNs and NAs *within* each type engaging in similar patterns of work. Both grades of nursing staff in primary wards spent a greater amount of time in direct patient care but less time in supplementary patient care and staff activities. Team and functional nursing staff spent more time with patients in domestic and administrative activities. The implications of these findings for the employment of NAs in care of the elderly wards are discussed.

This study comparing the work of nurses and auxiliaries raises many fundamental issues. Based on very rigorous data collection methods, it demonstrates that there are few great differences between the amount of care provided by these two groups. But on primary nursing wards it appears that more direct care is provided overal, compared with other organisational types, and it is done in collaboration within the team. It is tempting to make value judgements about the outcomes of these work patterns but very challenging to demonstrate differences. However it is noteworthy that the predominant ethos of the nursing wards pervades the whole team, where everyone gives priority to 'useful' patient-oriented activities. This study demonstrates that systematic observation and description of work patterns can be illuminating.

Quelle: *Nursing times* 1993 (89) 38

Try to answer the following questions about the text.

Exercise

1. *contribution* in line 2 means:
   a) contradiction
   b) participation
   c) respect
   d) defence

2. *perform* in line 4/5 means:
   a) to demonstrate
   b) to show
   c) to model
   d) to carry out

3. *randomly* in line 8/9 means:
   a) eventually
   b) every now and then
   c) accidentally
   d) deliberately

4. *implication* in line 22 means:
   a) meaning
   b) significance
   c) involvement
   d) conclusion

5. *fundamental issues* in line 26/27 means:
   a) basic
   b) most important subjects
   c) questions
   d) great problems

6. *collaboration* in line 34 means:
   a) betrayal
   b) agreement
   c) cooperation
   d) sharing

7. *outcome* in line 36 means:
   a) refuge
   b) result
   c) aim
   d) exit

8. *predominant* in line 39 means:
   a) first class
   b) leading
   c) outstanding
   d) suppressing

9. *pervade* in line 40 means:
   a) to imply
   b) to implicate
   c) to pervert
   d) to influence

11.2 Organization Types for Delivering a Nursing Service

Information

A) Task allocation or functional nursing

Nurses are allotted responsibility for carrying out delegated tasks common to all patients. It is a way of organizing staff to ensure that the minimum standard of physical care is achieved for all patients. However, care can be fragmented and does not incorporate the individual's comprehensive needs for nursing.

B) Team nursing

Team nursing is based on the belief that a small group of nurses working together led by one nurse, can give better care than they can if they work individually. It uses the skills of all team members so that the client gets the best care available. There are three prerequisites for team nursing:
- Each team is led by a registered nurse, who must have leadership and management skills;
- There must be effectivly written and spoken communication;
- The style of management must support the role of the team leader.

The team can choose a number of ways for the organization of its client's care on a daily basis, and there is flexibility in the size of the team, the caseload, and the time-span of the caseload.

C) Primary nursing

Primary nursing is described as a professional model of practice, in which a qualified nurse is responsible and accountable for the nursing care of a caseload of patients, for the entire duration of their care in that particular setting (for instance, ward, group home, own home). The principles of primary nursing are;
- The allocation and acceptance of individual responsibility and accountability for decision-making to one individual nurse;
- One nurse responsible for the coordination and quality of care administered to a group of patients 24 hours a day, 7 days a week.

The values underpinning primary nursing, centre on the belief that the nurse-patient relationship is therapeutic. It provides an environment and philosophy in which nurses can achieve maximum potential in patient centred care.

To which organizational types do the following descriptions belong?   *Exercise*

1. ... a small team of nurses is responsible and accountable for its group of patients during the whole of the patient's hospital stay.

2. ... the individual receives total daily care from one nurse, who has the freedom (autonomy) to carry out this practice.

3. ... one nurse does all the dressings or the drug rounds, another nurse carries out all the patients' vital observations.

Quelle: *Approaches to nursing care, issues in nursing and health*, Royal college of nursing, Jan. 1996

Match the following English words from the text in 11.2 with their German translation:

d) allocation	... 4.	aufnehmen, enthalten
e) functional nursing	... 5.	zu bewältigende Arbeit
f) to allot	... 6.	Vorbedingung, Voraussetzung
g) to incorporate	... 7.	untermauern
h) prerequisite	... 8.	beruhen auf
i) caseload	... 9.	Zuteilung, Zuweisung
j) particular setting	... 10.	Funktionspflege
k) underpinning	... 11.	zuweisen, verteilen
l) to centre	... 12.	Milieu, Umgebung, Umwelt
m) environment	... 13.	umschriebener Rahmen, Umfeld

ADDRESSOGRAPH LABEL

Admission Date: / /	
Age:	
Marital Status:	
Occupation:	
Religion:	
Likes to be referred to as:	

NEXT OF KIN

Name:	
Adress:	
Relationship:	
Tel. No. Home:	
Work:	
Children (if any):	
Meaningful Others:	
Informed of Admission	Yes/No
Notify at night	Yes/No
GP Name:	
Address:	
	Type of admission: Routine/Emergency
Telephone No:	
Room No.	Name:

PAST MEDICAL HISTORY

ALLERGIES

PREVIOUS ANAESTHETIC PROBLEMS

REASON FOR ADMISSION

OPERATION

Date / /	
Consent form seen:	Yes/No

PREMEDICATION

DRUGS CURRENTLY USED

DRUGS RECENTLY USED

NURSING OBSERVATIONS ON ADMISSION

Temp.:	Pulse:	Resp.:
B.P.:	Weight:	
Urine:		
Consultant:		

NUTRITION

Normal diet:

Special diet:

Alcohol

TEETH

Dentures:

Brace:

Crowns:

Other Problems:

ELIMINATION

Urinary Problems:

Menstruation:

Bowels: Daily/More Often

Problems?

SKIN CONDITION

Good .... Yes/No

Broken areas: .... Yes/No

Rashes .... Yes/No

Bruises: .... Yes/No

MOBILITY

Self care .... Yes/No

Aids used .... Yes/No

Help required .... Yes/No

BREATHING

Problems .... Yes/No

Details:

Smoker .... Yes/No

Type: Amount:

SLEEP PATTERN

Problems:

No. hours:

Sedation:

SIGHT

Good .... Yes/No

Glasses   Lenses:

HEARING

Good .... Yes/No

Problems Right:

Problems Left:

SPEECH

Impairment:

Language difficulty:

EMOTIONAL ATTITUDE

Patient's perception of illness

Good/Bad

RECENT LIFE CRISIS

MAINTAINING SAFE ENVIRONMENT

Alert: Confused:

OTHER RELEVANT COMMENTS

HOME CONDITIONS

SPIRITUAL NEEDS

Communion etc.

VALUABLES

With Patient   Yes/No

Nurses Custody   Yes/No

Detail:

ARRANGEMENTS/AFTERCARE

Date of Discharge: /   /

Relatives informed: Yes/No

Transport arranged: Yes/No

Doctor's letter:

TTO's: OPA:

NURSE ASSESSOR

Name: (CAPITALS)

Date:

11.3 Applying the Nursing Process

Information

The nursing process is a systematic, problem-solving approach of care-giving. Though it consists of several, subsequent steps, it is not a hierarchy but an cyclical process. In principle, there is an agreement regarding the relevant steps, though they are organized in four to five and six levels. The following is a five-step-approach common in the USA.

Assessment

Assessment is the collecting of all relevant information and data to enable the nurse to determine the patient's status and nursing needs. Nurses can gather information from written resources, during the admission or nursing interview, by physical assessment with measuring data, examining and observing the patient, etc.
Different pre-printed assessment preforma can help to record and organize the data.

Diagnosis

During diagnosis the nurse analyses the gathered data to identify the specific problems and resources of a patient. They form the basis for the plan of care.
As an attempt to standardize nursing diagnosis the NANDA (North American Nursing Diagnosis Association) developed a classification. It is called NANDA Taxonomy and is organized by the model of "human response patterns". The corresponding European organization is the ENDA (European Nursing Diagnosis Association).

Planning

Planning integrates various actions according to the client's individual needs of care. Thus the nurse sets priorities and establishes expected outcomes also defined as goals or aims of care. Furthermore the nurse chooses nursing actions or interventions suitable to solve the patient's problems and achieve the goals. The determined interventions are recorded in a care plan.

Implementation

Implementation means the phase of putting the care plan into action, i.e. to perform the prescribed nursing actions and to assess the effects on the patient.

Evaluation

Evaluation means to check whether the goals of care have been achieved. The nurse reviews the situation to see whether or not the problems still exist or new ones have developed. Evaluation may result in a completely new circle of the nursing process or in modifying single components of it.

11.4 Phrasal Verbs

Phrasal verbs are verbs followed by prepositions as mentioned in 7.8 or an adverbial particle. In everyday conversation the use of phrasal verbs instead of more formal verbs is quite common. So make another exercise so you can understand what your patient says.

Match the phrasal verbs in the following sentences with the appropriate meaning: *Exercise*

1. In the morning I always *bring up* a lot of phlegm.

   _____

2. Just the smell of it *turns* my stomach *over* and sometimes I *bring back* the whole food.

   _____   _____

3. The doctor told me to *leave* coffee *out* of my diet, but I like it too much.

   _____

4. Since I have arthritis I am not able to *do up* my shirt.

   _____

5. I can't *get through* that again.

   _____

6. Sorry, I didn't want to *put* you *out*.

   _____

7. Maybe her intentions are good. But I can't *make* her *out*.

   _____

8. Yes, when I try to *get up*, I nearly *break down*. But I'll *come round* soon.

_____   _____   _____

9. Maybe I've *put on* some kilos since I have quitted smoking, but now I'm sick I'll *take them off* soon enough.

_____   _____

10. I'm still very *cut up* about these news.

_____

11. I felt very sick, but now I *get on* very well.

_____

to omit   to bear it   to understand   to collapse   to gain weight   to be very upset
to expectorate   to vomit   to button   to leave the bed   to regain consciousness   to feel
queasy/sick   to irritate   to improve   to reduce weight

11.5 Translation

Exercise

Translate the following questions you might ask the patient:

1. Wer sind Ihre nächsten Angehörigen/für Sie wichtige Bezugspersonen?

_____

2. Wie empfinden Sie Ihre Situation/Krankheit?

_____

3. Können Sie Ihre Schmerzen beschreiben? Wo haben Sie Schmerzen? Seit wann haben Sie Schmerzen?

_____

4. Wobei kann ich Ihnen helfen? Was kann ich für Sie tun?

_____

5. Wie sind Sie bisher zu Hause zurechtgekommen?

_____

11.6 When- und If-Sätze mit Ereignissen in der Zukunft (when I do ... /if I do ...)

A) Betrachten Sie folgendes Beispiel: *Grammar*

Nurse: When do you want get up today?
Wann wollen Sie heute aufstehen?

Patient: I'll get up when the pain goes off.
Ich werde aufstehen, wenn die Schmerzen nachlassen.

"I'll get up when the pain goes off" ist ein zweiteiliger Satz. "I'll get up" bildet den Hauptsatz und "when the pain goes off" den *When*-Satz. Dieser Satz beschreibt ein Geschehen in der Zukunft, dennoch werden in Sätzen mit dem Element *when* die Formen *will* oder *going to* nicht benutzt. Stattdessen wird eine Gegenwartsform verwendet, im Allgemeinen *simple present* (I do).

- I'll ring you up when I leave the ward >> *nicht* "when I will leave"
- When you see him, he'll tell you about it >> *nicht* "when you will see him"

Das Gleiche gilt für entsprechende Sätze mit
- *while – after – before – until/till – as soon as*

- Her sister will look after the children while Mrs Fields is in hospital.
- Before you leave, you must drink a cup of tea with me.
- I'm afraid you'll have to wait until the doctor comes back.

B) Um auszudrücken, dass ein erstes Ereignis/Geschehen vor dem zweiten beendet sein wird, kann man nach *when/after/until etc.* auch das *present perfect* verwenden.

- When I've weighed Mrs Snow, you can get the scales.
- Don't disturb Mrs Miller while her husband is here. Wait until he has gone.

Oft ist es möglich sowohl *simple present* als auch *present perfect* zu verwenden:

- I'll tell the children as soon as they arrive.
- I'll tell the children as soon as they have arrived.
- You'll feel better after you have something to eat.
- You'll feel better after you have had something to eat.

C) Nach *if* in Bezug auf zukünftige Ereignisse wird ebenfalls das *present simple* (I do) anstatt einer Zukunftsform verwendet:

- If Bob leaves immediately, he'll catch the 6.30 bus >> *nicht* "if he will leave"
- He won't catch it if he doesn't hurry >> *nicht* "if he won't hurry"

Die unterschiedliche Verwendung von *when* und *if* muss dabei berücksichtigt werden.
When wird eingesetzt, wenn Ereignisse *sicher* stattfinden werden:

- I'm going to work this morning. When I go working, I'll meet my workmates.

If wird eingesetzt, wenn Ereignisse *möglicherweise* stattfinden werden:

- If it rains this afternoon, I'll go to the cinema instead of the park.
- Stay at home if you don't feel better tomorrow.

Exercise

A) Put the verbs into the correct form.

1. Everyone _____ (be) very glad if he _____ (survive) the accident.

2. When Mrs Fields _____ (get) indigestion, a bland diet _____ (bring) her relief.

3. As soon as the urgent laboratory results _____ (arrive) call the doctor.

4. I'm not tired enough. If I _____ (go) to bed now, I _____ (not sleep).

5. Mr Stout _____ (be discharged) as soon as his leg ulcer _____ (heal).

B) Choose if or when.

6. You'll hurt each other _____ you're not careful.

7. I'll go to the new patient later. _____ I'm there I'll take her temperature.

8. _____ you use so much gauze, we'll run out.

C) Make one sentence from two sentences.

9. We'll receive the last result of the X-ray tomorrow. Then we'll talk about your treatment.

_____ as soon as _____

10. You must have a medical check-up. Then you take the job.

Before _____

11.7 Determining Nursing Interventions

For each problem and goal/aim of care listed below translate the possible nursing actions.   *Exercise*

	Problems	Aims	Prescribed Care
1.	Anxiety re pending surgery	will have an understanding of procedure and outcome	* teach the patient what to expect pre and postoperative, e.g. about drains, catheters, deep breathing exercises and so on _____ _____ * Assess areas of anxiety the patient may have and discuss them _____ _____
2.	High risk for alterations in skin integrity (pressure ulcers)	will maintain intact skin	* assess skin integrity with each position change _____ _____ * develop a turning schedule and turn 2 hourly _____ _____

	Problems	Aims	Prescribed Care
3.	Alteration of the body image related to breast cancer surgery	will adapt to her changing body image and will keep a feeling of self-esteem	* Ermutige die Patientin ihre Gefühle der Angst, der Furcht vor Verstümmelung und vor Ablehnung auszudrücken _____ * Ermutige und unterstütze die Patienten ihren Körper/ihre Narben anzusehen und zu berühren _____
4.	Impaired communication related to aphasia	will develop communication styles which enable him to express needs	* Beschaffe Hilfsmittel zur Verständigung (z.B. Tafel, Bilder) _____ * Bleibe gelassen und unterstützend, lass dem Patienten genug Zeit zu antworten und zu sprechen

11.8 Reaching towards Wholeness

The Concept of Holistic Nursing

Text

Holism is derived from the Greek *holos* meaning 'whole', and is in contrast to the modern daily experience of life which tends toward fragmentation, with threats to autonomous living which may lead to illness if the level of fragmentation becomes too great. Holistic philosophy proposes that the uncompromised individual always responds as a unified whole. A holistic approach places importance on understanding the multiple dimensions of human existence and experience and finds it inappropriate to consider only one aspect, such as a physical symptom, an emotion, or a response to an environmental stimulus, apart from the complete context.

The Holistic Nursing Association in the UK believes that everyone can move towards greater wellness when the conditions around and within them are valued and upheld. Holistic nursing recognizes that health proceeds from a balance of our physical, spiritual, psychological and social needs. Our wholeness is dependent on our relationship to each other, our environment and that what gives our lives meaning. Holistic nursing begins with an open mind and willingness to explore the potential for personal growth, health and well-being for ourselves and others. Holistic nursing seeks to be instrumental in creating a healing opportunity not only for the patient but for the person of the nurse.

Holistic nursing can enable the nurse to achieve balance and well-being while integrating life, work and health to reach optimum human potential, even at a time of challenge and uncertainty. ...

Holism, as 'whole-person care', is therefore not about setting up a tension or alternative opposition to traditional modalities of healing. It is to broaden, enhance and complement these approaches.

Quelle: *European Nurse* 1996 (1) 4

Are the following statements about the text true or false?

		true	false	*Exercise*
1.	A fragmentary lifestyle can work as a pathogenic influence and may cause diseases.	❏	❏	
2.	A holistic approach investigates various aspects of living separately.	❏	❏	
3.	Wellness according to the holistic philosophy can be achieved by everyone under appropriate circumstances.	❏	❏	
4.	Holistic nursing as the healing power is particularly important for the patient.	❏	❏	
5.	Holistic nursing also includes traditional methods of caring.	❏	❏	

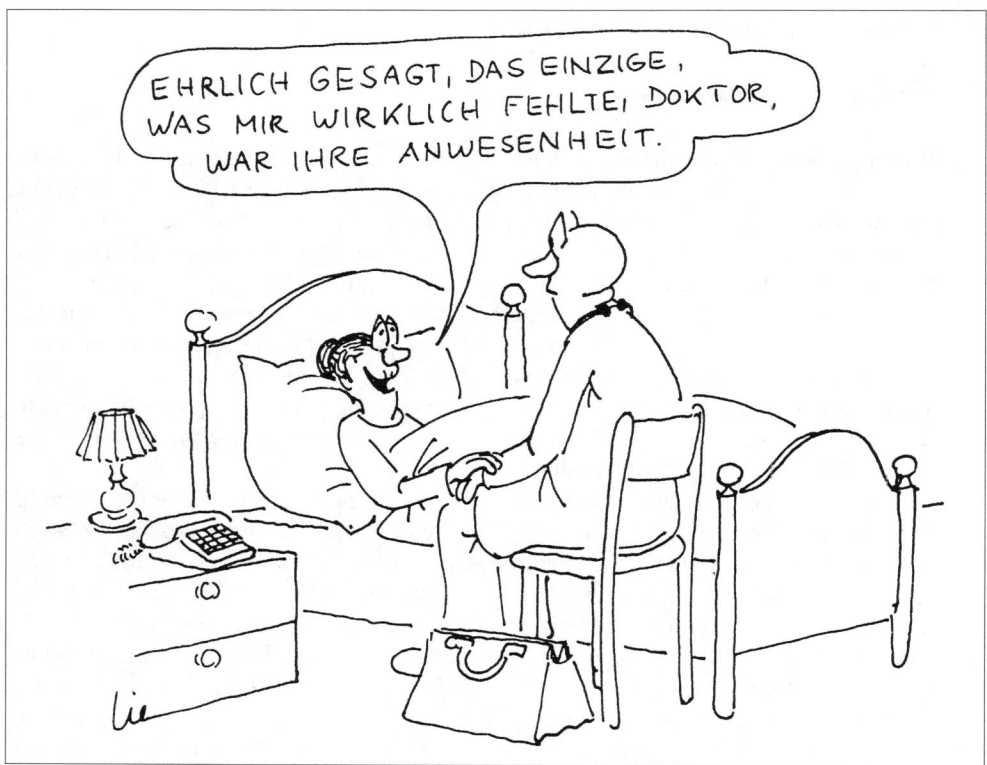

Quelle: Löwensteiner Cartoon Service (Hrsg.): Dr. med. Ironicus. Thieme, Stuttgart 1994 (S. 75)

11.9 Complementary Therapy

Puzzle

The WHO defined complementary therapies as those which can work alongside and in conjunction with orthodox medical treatment. A lot of nurses show interest in those methods and attend courses to extend their experience and potentials. Though, complementary therapies are not synonymous with holism and should be viewed as supplementary to both conventional and holistic approaches.

Try to fit the following definitions for types of complementary therapies into the diagram.

1. A system of medicine in which a disease is treated by giving extremely small amounts of a substance that causes the disease.

2. To press and rub someone's body with hands to reduce pain and tension.

3. The use of hypnosis to treat emotional problems, or fears, etc.

4. To use one's natural ability to cure people.

5. The method of listening to people and giving them support with their problems and in developing their inner strengths.

6. A treatment in which fine needles are inserted to specific points on the body.

7. Another word for complementary (medicine).

8. The treatment of illness by talking to someone or discussing their problems.

9. A medicine working with extracts from plants.

10. A therapy based on massage of reflex points of the feet corresponding with body parts and organs.

11. A way of treating physical problems by moving and pressing muscles and bones.

Appendix A   Irregular Verbs

Verb (base)	Imperfect (past tense)	zweites Partizip (-ed participle)	Bedeutung
awake	awoke/awaked	awoken/awaked	aufwachen
be	was/were	been	sein
bear	bore	borne	tragen
beat	beat	beaten	schlagen
become	became	become	werden
beget	begot	begotten	zeugen
begin	began	begun	beginnen
bend	bent	bent	beugen
bet	bet/betted	bet/betted	wetten
bid	bade/bid	bid/bidden	wünschen
bind	bound	bound	binden
bite	bit	bitten	beißen
bleed	bled	bled	bluten
blow	blew	blown	blasen
break	broke	broken	brechen
bring	brought	brought	bringen
build	built	built	bauen
burn	burnt/burned	burnt/burned	brennen
burst	burst	burst	bersten
buy	bought	bought	kaufen
cast	cast	cast	werfen
catch	caught	caught	fangen
choose	chose	chosen	auswählen
cling	clung	clung	sich festklammern
come	came	come	kommen
cost	cost	cost	kosten
creep	crept	crept	kriechen
cut	cut	cut	schneiden
deal	dealt	dealt	handeln
dig	dug	dug	graben
do	did	done	tun
draw	drew	drawn	zeichnen, ziehen
dream	dreamt/dreamed	dreamt/dreamed	träumen
drink	drank	drunk	trinken
drive	drove	driven	fahren
eat	ate	eaten	essen
fall	fell	fallen	fallen
feed	fed	fed	ernähren, füttern
feel	felt	felt	fühlen
fight	fought	fought	streiten, kämpfen
find	found	found	finden
flee	fled	fled	flüchten
fly	flew	flown	fliegen
forbid	forbad(e)	forbidden	verbieten
forget	forgot	forgotten	vergessen
freeze	froze	frozen	frieren, einfrieren
get	got	got	bekommen

Verb (base)	Imperfect (past tense)	zweites Partizip (-ed participle)	Bedeutung
give	gave	given	geben
go	went	gone	gehen
grow	grew	grown	wachsen
hang	hung	hung	hängen
have	had	had	haben
hear	heard	heard	hören
heave	heaved/hove	heaved/hove	heben
hide	hid	hidden	verbergen
hit	hit	hit	treffen
hold	held	held	halten
hurt	hurt	hurt	verletzen, Schmerz zufügen
keep	kept	kept	behalten
kneel	knelt/knelled	knelt/knelled	knien
knit	knit/knitted	knit/knitted	stricken
know	knew	known	wissen
lay	laid	laid	legen
lead	led	led	führen
lean	leant/leaned	leant/leaned	lehnen
learn	learnt/learned	learnt/learned	lernen
leave	left	left	verlassen, lassen
lend	lent	lent	leihen
let	let	let	lassen, vermieten
lie	lay	lain	liegen
light	lit/lighted	lit/lighted	anzünden, beleuchten
lose	lost	lost	verlieren
make	made	made	machen
mean	meant	meant	meinen
meet	met	met	treffen
overcome	overcame	overcome	überwältigen, überwinden
pay	paid	paid	bezahlen
put	put	put	legen, setzen, stellen
read	read	read	lesen
redo	redid	redone	wiederholen
ride	rode	ridden	fahren, reiten
ring	rang	rung	läuten, klingeln
rise	rose	risen	ansteigen
run	ran	run	rennen
saw	sawed	sawn/sawed	sägen
say	said	said	sagen
see	saw	seen	sehen
seek	sought	sought	suchen
sell	sold	sold	verkaufen
send	sent	sent	versenden, verschicken
set	set	set	stellen, setzen
sew	sewed	sewn/sewed	nähen
shake	shook	shaken	schütteln
shed	shed	shed	Blut, Tränen vergießen

Verb (base)	Imperfect (past tense)	zweites Partizip (-ed participle)	Bedeutung
shine	shone/shined	shone/shined	scheinen
shoot	shot	shot	schießen
show	showed	shown	zeigen
shut	shut	shut	schließen
sing	sang	sung	singen
sink	sank	sunk	sinken
sit	sat	sat	sitzen
slay	slew	slain	töten
sleep	slept	slept	schlafen
slide	slid	slid	gleiten
smell	smelt/smelled	smelt/smelled	riechen
speak	spoke	spoken	sprechen
spell	spelt/spelled	spelt/spelled	buchstabieren
spend	spent	spent	ausgeben, verbringen
spill	spilt/spilled	spilt/spilled	verschütten
spit	spat/spit	spat/spit	spucken
spread	spread	spread	verbreiten, ausbreiten
spring	sprang	sprung	springen
stand	stood	stood	stehen
steal	stole	stolen	stehlen
stick	stuck	stuck	anheften, ankleben
sting	stung	stung	stechen
stink	stank	stunk	stinken
strike	struck	struck	schlagen, treffen, stoßen
sweat	sweat/sweated	sweat/sweated	schwitzen
sweep	swept	swept	fegen
swell	swelled	swollen/swelled	schwellen
swim	swam	swum	schwimmen
swing	swung	swung	schwingen
take	took	taken	nehmen
teach	taught	taught	lehren, unterrichten
tear	tore	torn	reißen
tell	told	told	erzählen, sagen
think	thought	thought	denken
throw	threw	thrown	werfen
understand	understood	understood	verstehen
unwind	unwound	unwound	abwickeln, entwirren
upset	upset	upset	aus der Fassung bringen
wake	woke/waked	woken/waked	wecken
wear	wore	worn	tragen (Kleidung)
weep	wept	wept	weinen
win	won	won	gewinnen
wind	wound	wound	winden
withhold	withheld	withheld	vorenthalten
withstand	withstood	withstood	standhalten, widerstehen
write	wrote	written	schreiben

Nutrition

There are several things that keep people healthy. One very important factor is a balanced diet. Different food contains different substances needed by the body. These substances are necessary for protection, construction of body cells and as an energy source.

function	substance	example
energy source	carbohydrates	fruit, grain
	proteins	fish, vegetables
	fats	peanuts, milk
protection	minerals	milk, eggs
	vitamins	oil, vegetables
construction	proteins	rice, potatoes
	minerals	cheese, meat

Vitamins are essential food factors. Their absence can cause various deficiency diseases. Here are examples of the main vitamins and some products in which they can be found.

vitamins	products
vitamin **A**/retinol	milk, carrots, tomatoes
vitamin **D**/**D2** ergocalciferol	fish, egg yolk
D3 cholecalciferol	produced by sunlight
vitamin **E**/tocopherol	wheat germ, butter
vitamin **K**/phytomenadione menaquinone	green vegetables meat
vitamin **B1**/thiamine	cereals, beans, nuts
B2/riboflavin	liver, milk, eggs
B6/pyridoxine	potatoes, eggs, fish
B12/cobalamin	liver, fish, eggs
vitamin **C**/ascorbic acid	citrus fruits, vegetables

Appendix C Vocabulary: English-German

Für alle Berufe gilt sowohl die männliche als auch die weibliche Form. Regelmäßig steht „(to)" hinter einem Wort, um damit anzugeben, dass es sich um ein Verb handelt. Die Übersetzung der Wörter bezieht sich in den meisten Fällen auf den Kontext dieses Buches.

English	German	English	German
A & E nurse	Krankenpfleger Erste Hilfe	admit (to)	aufnehmen (in ein-Krankenhaus
abbreviation	Abkürzung	adoption	Adoption
abdomen	Bauch	advantage	Vorteil
abdominal	Bauch betreffend	affect (to)	beeinflussen
ability	Fertigkeit, Fähigkeit	afloat	treibend
abnormality	Abweichung	ageing population	Überalterung
abscess	Abszess, Eitergeschwür	agreement	Übereinstimmung, Vereinbarung
abuse	Missbrauch		
access	Zugang	ahead	vor, voran
accident and emergency	Erste Hilfe	ailment	Krankheit
		aim	Ziel, Absicht
accidental	zufällig, versehentlich	air passages	Luftwege
accomodate (to)	helfen, unterbringen	air way	Luftwege
according to	gemäß, entsprechend	alike	ebenso
account for (to)	erklären, der Grund sein für	allegation	Behauptung
		alleviate (to)	lindern
account (to take into)	berücksichtigen	allow (to)	erlauben, gestatten
accountable	verantwortlich	alteration	Veränderung
accurately	präzise, genau	alternately	abwechselnd
accusation	Beschuldigung, Anklage	although	obwohl
		altruistic	uneigennützig
achieve (to)	erreichen	AMA	gegen den Rat der Ärzte
acromion	Akromion		
acronym	Akronym	ambiguous	zweideutig
Act	Gesetz	ambulant	ambulant
acupuncture	Akkupunktur	amendment	Änderung, Besserung
acute conditions	akute Konditionen	amniocentesis	Fruchblasenpunktion
add (to)	hinzuzählen, hinzufügen	amnion	Fruchtblase
		amniotic fluid	Fruchtwasser
address (to)	richten auf	amount	Menge
adhesive plaster	Heftpflaster	ancillary	Neben-, Hilfs-
adjust (to)	einstellen, regulieren	ankle	Knöchel
administer (to)	verabreichen	antacid	Antiazidum
administration	Verabreichung, Verwaltung	antidote	Gegengift
		antiseptic	antiseptisch
administrator	Verwalter, Leiter	antivenom	Gegengift
admire (to)	bewundern	anxiety	Angst, Besorgnis
admission	Aufnahme	apathy	Apathie, Lustlosigkeit
		apparent	offensichtlich, klar, scheinbar

English	German	English	German
appear	erscheinen	bargain (to)	verhandeln
application	Anwendung	bath blanket	Handtuch (USA)
approach	Annäherung, Ansatz	bathe (to)	baden
appropriate	richtig, geeignet	bathroom	Badezimmer
approve (to)	einverstanden sein	beat (to)	schlagen
approximately	circa	bedclothes	Bettzeug
arise (to)	entstehen	bedcradle	Bettbahre
arm hole	Ärmelloch	bedpan	Bettpfanne
armpit	Achsel	bedside table	Nachtschränkchen
arrange (to)	ordnen, vereinbaren	bedsore	wundgelegene Stelle
arrangement	Vereinbarung, Anord-nung	behave (to)	verhalten
		bahaviour	Verhalten
arrest (to)	hemmen	belief	Glaube
arrhythmia	Arrhythmie	bell push	Klingelknopf
arterial	Arterien betreffend	belly	Bauch
artery	Schlagader	bend over (to)	vornüber beugen
artificial ventilation	künstliche Beatmung	benefit	Vorteil, Nutzen
a.s.a.p.	so schnell wie möglich	bereavement	Trauerfall
aspersion	abfällige Bemerkung	big toe	großer Zeh
assess (to)	beurteilen	bikini cut	Bikinischnitt
assessment	Einschätzung, Feststel-lung	biliary colics	Gallenkolik
		bilirubin	Gallenfarbstoff
association	Vereinigung	BKA	Unterschenkelampu-tation
assurance	Versicherung		
assure (to)	versichern	bladder	Blase
ASU	Aufnahme Urinunter-suchung	blanket	Decke
		blister	(Wasser-, Blut-) Blase
attach (to)	befestigen	blood disorder	Blutkrankheit
attempt (to)	versuchen	blood loss	Blutverlust
attend (to)	anwesend sein, behan-deln	blood pressure (BP)	Blutdruck
		blood sample	Blutprobe
attendance	Behandlung	blood sugar level	Blutzuckerspiegel
attention	Aufmerksamkeit	blouse	Bluse
attitude	Haltung, Standpunkt	blur (to)	verwischen, verschlei-ern
audit (to)	prüfen, belegen		
aural thermometer	Ohrthermometer	body fluids	Körperflüssigkeiten
auscultation	Abhören	body-image	Körperbild
autoimmune disease	Autoimmunerkran-kung	body language	Körpersprache
		body temperature	Körpertemperatur
available	verfügbar	body tissue	Körpergewebe
avoid (to)	vermeiden, verhüten	boil	Furunkel
axilla	Achsel	boil (to)	kochen
		boiling point	Siedepunkt
back	Rücken	bone marrow	Knochenmark
back rub	Rückenabreibung	bother (to)	belästigen, stören
back shift	Spätdienst	bottle-feed (to)	aus der Flasche ernähren
back up (to)	unterstützen		
backwards	rückwärts	bowel	Darm
bandage	Verband	bra	BH
bar	Stock, Stange	bradycardia	Bradykardie

English	German	English	German
brain	Gehirn	caution	Vorsicht
breach (to)	durchbrechen	cavity	Höhle, Höhlung
breast-feed (to)	stillen	central nervous system	zentrales Nervensystem
breath	Atem	tem	tem
breech presentation	Steißlage	cereals	Getreideprodukte
briefs	Slip (UK)	challenge	Herausforderung
broaden a scope (to)	den Blick erweitern	change (to)	wechseln, umziehen
bronchoscopy	Bronchoskopie	character	Kennzeichen, Art
bruise	blauer Fleck	charge (to be in)	verantwortlich sein
buck	Dollar	charge nurse	Pflegeleiter
built-in	eingebaut	charitable	gütig, wohltätig
bum	Hintern	charity	Barmherzigkeit, Güte
burn (to)	verbrennen	chart	Kurve, Fieberkurve
burning feeling	Brennen	chat	Plauderei
business department	Finanzabteilung	cheap	preiswert, billig
buttocks	Gesäß	checklist	Kontroll-Liste
button	Knopf	check-up	medizinische Untersu-
button (to)	knöpfen		chung
byproduct	Abfallprodukt	chemical plant	Chemiebetrieb
		chemist	Drogist
cable	Telegramm	chest	Brust, Brustkorb
Caesarean section	Kaiserschnitt	chew (to)	kauen
calcaneus	Fersenbein	CHF	Herzinsuffizienz
calculus	Stein	chill	Schüttelfrost
calf	Wade	chill (to)	abkühlen
call for (to)	fordern, verlangen	choke (to)	würgen, ersticken
cancer	Krebs	circulation	Blutkreislauf
candidosis	Candidose	circumcise (to)	beschneiden
cap	Haube	circumstances	Umstände
capable (to be)	in der Lage (sein)	CK	Kontrolle
capital letter	Großbuchstabe	claim (to)	behaupten, beanspru-
carbohydrate metabo-	Kohlehydratstoff-		chen
lism	wechsel	clap	Gonorrhoe
cardiac arrest	Herzstillstand	clarity	Klarheit
cardiac massage	Herzmassage	clavicle	Schlüsselbein
cardigan	Strickjacke	cleanse (to)	reinigen
cardiology	Kardiologie	clear	hell, klar
careful(ly)	vorsichtig	clinical experience	klinische Erfahrung
care of the elderly	Altenpflege	cloth	Tuch, Verband
carotid artery	Halsschlagader	COAD	chronisch-obstruktive
carpal	Handwurzelknochen		Atemwegserkran-
carry out (to)	ausführen		kung
cartilage	Knorpel	coagulation defect	Gerinnungsstörung
case	Fall	coated tablet	Dragee
case history	Anamnese, Kranken-	cobra	Kobra, Brillenschlange
	geschichte	coccyx	Steißbein
cast light on (to)	verdeutlichen	coincidence	Zufall, Fügung
casualty	Opfer	collaboration	Zusammenarbeit
cause	Ursache, Grund	collapse (to)	kollabieren
caustic	ätzend, kaustisch	collect (to)	sammeln

English	German	English	German
colon	Dickdarm	conjunction	Verbindung, Zusammentreffen
colostrum	Vormilch		
comfort	Komfort, Trost	conjunctiva	Bindehaut
comfort (to)	trösten	connect (to)	verbinden, anschließen
command (to)	befehlen		
commence (to)	beginnen	consensus	Übereinstimmung, Konsens
comment	Bemerkung, Kommentar		
		consent (to)	zustimmen
commission (to)	beauftragen, in Auftrag geben	consequences	Folgen
		consider (to)	berücksichtigen, bedenken, betrachten als
common(ly)	gemeinsam, allgemein, weitverbreitet		
		considerable	ansehnlich, beträchtlich
community	Gemeinde, Allgemeinheit		
		consist of (to)	bestehen aus
community medicine	Gemeindepflege	construction	Aufbau
compel (to)	zwingen	consultant	Facharzt
complain (to)	klagen, sich beschweren	consultative	beratend
		consume (to)	konsumieren, verzehren, verbrauchen
complaint	Beschwerde		
complementary	ergänzend	consumption	Verbrauch, Schwindsucht
compliance	Gehorsam		
compound fracture	komplizierter Bruch	contain (to)	enthalten
comprehensive	umfassend	contemptuous	geringschätzig, verächtlich
computerised event recorder	computergesteuerte Aufzeichnung		
		contents	Inhalt
conceive (to)	schwanger werden, empfangen	content with	zufrieden mit
		continue (to)	fortsetzen
conception	Befruchtung, Empfängnis	contract (to)	zusammenziehen
		contraction	Wehe
concern	Besorgnis	contracture	Kontraktur
concerned with (to be)	zu tun haben mit	contribute (to)	beitragen
conciseness	Präzision, Exaktheit	contribution	Mitwirkung, Beteiligung
conclude (to)	beenden, folgern		
conclusive	überzeugend, schlüssig	control (to)	kontrollieren, überwachen
condition	Kondition, Bedingung	controversial	kontrovers, umstritten
conduct (to)	führen, leiten	convalescence	Rekonvaleszenz, Genesung
conduction	Leitung		
condyle	Gelenkkopf	convert (to)	konvertieren, umwandeln
confidentiality	Vertraulichkeit		
confined to bed (to be)	das Bett hüten müssen	convince (to)	überzeugen
		cool (to)	kühlen
confirm a diagnosis (to)	eine Diagnose stellen	cornea	Hornhaut
		corresponding	entsprechend, in Einklang mit
confirmation	Bestätigung		
conflict (to)	widersprechen	costal	kostal, Rippen betreffend
confused	verwirrt		
congenital	angeboren	counselling	Beratung

English	German	English	German
counteract (to)	entgegenwirken, neutralisieren	dental surgery	Zahn- und Kieferchirurgie
course of a disease	Krankheitsverlauf	depend on (to)	abhängig sein von
cover (to)	bedecken	deprive of (to)	entziehen, vorenthalten
co-worker	Kollege		
cranium	Schädel	derive (to)	ableiten (von), gewinnen, erhalten
creature	Geschöpf, Tier		
crib	Kinderbettchen	dermatitis	Hautentzündung
cripple	Invalide, Krüppel	dermatology	Dermatologie
critically (ill)	ernsthaft (krank)	derogatory	abschätzig, abfällig
cure	Behandlung, Heilverfahren	description	Beschreibung
		desire	Wunsch, Verlangen
current	aktuell, Strömung, Strom	destroy (to)	zerstören
		determine (to)	feststellen, bestimmen
cut	Schnitt		
cut (to)	schneiden	development	Entwicklung
cute	niedlich, schlau	diaphragm	Zwerchfell, Diaphragma
cutting	scharf, Schnitt, Ausschnitt		
		diarrhoea	Diarrhoe
cyclical	zyklisch	diastolic pressure	distolischer Druck
		dietary department	Zentralküche
damaged	beschädigt	difficulties in	Schwierigkeiten mit
data	Informationen	digestive tract	Verdauungstrakt
D & C	Erweiterung und Ausschabung	digestive tube	Verdauungstrakt
		dilate (to)	ausdehnen, erweitern
deafness	Taubheit	dilatation (UK)	Erweiterung, Ausdehnung
debate	Diskussion, Debatte		
decade	Jahrzehnt	dilation (USA)	Erweiterung, Ausdehnung
decision	Entscheidung, Entschluss		
		disadvantage	Nachteil
decrease	Abnahme, Rückgang	disappearance	Verschwinden, Schwinden
deem (to)	erachten, halten für		
defecation	Reinigung, Darmentleerung	disaster	Unglück, Katastrophe
		discharge	Ausscheidung, Absonderung, Entlassung
defect	Störung		
deficiency	Mangel, Unvollkommenheit	discolour (to)	verfärben
		discomfort	Beschwerde (körperl.), Unannehmlichkeit
deflate (to)	ablassen (Luft)		
degree	Maß, Abschluss	discourage (to)	abraten, abhalten, entmutigen
dehydration	Austrocknung		
delegate (to)	delegieren, übertragen	dislocation	Verrenkung, Verlagerung
deliberate	bewusst, absichtlich	dislodge (to)	lösen, verdrängen
deliver (to)	liefern, entbinden	disorder	Unordnung, Störung, Erkrankung
delivery	Zustellung, Entbindung		
		disorderly	nachlässig
demand (to)	fordern, verlangen	dispense (to)	austeilen, dispensieren
demoralized	entmutigt	disposable	Wegwerf-
denial	Ablehnung	dissatisfied	unzufrieden
dental health	Zahngesundheit		

English	German	English	German
distinction	Unterschied, Auszeichnung	efficacy	Wirksamkeit
distinguish (to)	unterscheiden, erkennen	eggcrate mattress	Schaumstoffmatratze
		egg yolk	Eidotter
distress	Sorge, Qual, Schmerz	elbow	Ellenbogen
district nurse	Fürsorgepfleger	elderly	ältere Leute, ältlich
disturbance	Störung, Behinderung, Verwirrung	electric current	Strom
		elevator	Aufzug
disturbed consciousness	Bewusstseinsstörung	elimination	Ausscheidung, Entfernung, Beseitigung
disturbing	störend, beunruhigend	elixir	Elixier
		embarrassing	peinlich
diversity	Verschiedenheit	embarrassment	Verlegenheit
divide (to)	teilen	embolism	Embolie
division of cells	Zellteilung	emergency	Notfall
dizziness	Schwindel	emergency department	Notaufnahme
DNR	nicht reanimieren		
DoH (Department of Health)	Gesundheitsamt	emesis basin	Brechschale
		emphasize (to)	betonen, hervorheben
domestic	häuslich, zum Haushalt gehörend	employ (to)	anstellen, beschäftigen, anwenden
domiciliary	Hausbesuch	endogenous	endogen
dosage	Dosierung, Dosis	enable (to)	befähigen
doubt	Zweifel	enema	Klistier
doubtful	zweifelhaft	enhance (to)	steigern, erhöhen
dress (to)	anziehen	enlargement	Vergrößerung, Erweiterung
draw up (to)	aufstellen, aufziehen		
drip	Tropfinfusion	enlightenment	Aufklärung, Erleuchtung
droplet method	Tropfenausbreitung		
drown (to)	ertränken	enrolled nurse (EN)	Pfleger 2. Grades
drug addict	Drogenabhängiger	ensure (to)	sicherstellen
drug round	Arzneimittelvergabe	ENT (ear-nose-throat)	HNO
dubious	zweifelhaft	entire	völlig, Gesamt-
due to	aufgrund, wegen	entry level	Zulassungsanforderungen
duodenum	Zwölffingerdarm		
duration	Dauer	episiotomy	Episiotomie
during	während	equipment	Material, Ausrüstung
dust	Staub	equity	Fairness, Billigkeit
dyspepsia	Dyspepsie	equivalent	gleichwertig, gleich
		eradicate (to)	ausrotten
early shift	Frühdienst	erase (to)	ausschaben
ease	Erleichterung, Linderung	establish (to)	gründen, einführen
		estimate (to)	schätzen
eavesdrop (to)	belauschen, lauschen	etiology	Ätiologie
eczema	Ekzem	evaluate (to)	bewerten, auswerten
edit (to)	herausgeben	evidence	Beweis
educational	Ausbildung betreffend	evolve (to)	entwickeln
educational experience	Ausbildungserfahrung	example	Beispiel
		exacerbation	Verschlechterung, Verschlimmerung
effective(ly)	effektiv, wirksam		

English	German	English	German
exceed (to)	überschreiten, übersteigen	fetus	Fötus
excess	Übermaß, Überschuss	fever	Fieber
excessive	übermäßig	fibre	Faser
excision	Ausschneiden, Entfernung	fibula	Wadenbein
		fifth (5th) toe	kleiner Zeh
exclusion	Ausschluss	findings	Befund
excrete (to)	ausscheiden, abscheiden	finish (to)	beenden, erledigen
		firm(ly)	fest, stabil, sicher
exercise	Übung	fit	Anfall
exert (to)	ausüben	flabbergasted	fassungslos
exhalation	Ausatmung	flow	Strom, Fluss, Menstruation
existence	Bestehen, Existenz	flu	Grippe
exogenous	exogen	fluff	Daunen, Flaum
expand (to)	ausdehnen	fluid	Flüssigkeit
expect (to)	erwarten	fluid intake	Flüssigkeitszufuhr
expectant	erwartungsvoll	fluid output	Flüssigkeitsausscheidung
expectorate (to)	aushusten		
expenditures	Ausgaben, Kosten	flush (to)	erröten, ausspülen
expiration	Ausatmung	focus (to)	fokussieren, konzentrieren
explain (to)	erklären		
explore (to)	erforschen, untersuchen	foetus	Fötus
		force (to)	zwingen
express (to)	ausdrücken	forceps delivery	Zangengeburt
expression	Ausdruck, Auspressen	forearm	Unterarm
expulsion	Austreibung	foreign body	Fremdkörper
		forefinger	Zeigefinger
factual	tatsächlich, sachlich	forward	vorwärts
failure	Versagen, Störung, Insuffizienz	fourth (4th) toe	vierter Zeh
		fracture	Bruch, Fraktur
faint	schwach, Ohnmacht	fragmented	in Teile zerlegt
faint (to)	ohnmächtig werden	freeze (to)	frieren, einfrieren
fairly	ziemlich	frequently	regelmäßig
fall ill (to)	krank werden	frightened	ängstlich, erschrocken
false	falsch, unwahr, fehlerhaft	fruit squash	Fruchtgetränk
		full stop	Punkt
fasten (to)	befestigen	fundamental issues	grundlegende Fragen
fatigue	Ermüdung, Erschöpfung	funding	Finanzierung
		fungus	Pilz, Schimmel
fear	Angst		
feature	Kennzeichen, Merkmal, Gesichtszug	gain (to)	gewinnen
		gallstones	Gallensteine
federal	föderativ, Bundes-	gangrene	Brand (Nekrose)
feeding cup	Schnabeltasse	gargle	Gurgeln, Gurgelwasser
feel queasy (to)	Übelkeit verspüren	garment	Kleidungsstück
Fellow	Mitglied einer Wissenschaftlichen Vereinigung	gastritis	Magenentzündung
		gastrointestinal	Magen-Darm-, gastrointestinal
femur	Oberschenkel (-knochen)	gather (to)	sammeln, versammeln
		gauze	Gaze, Mull

English	German	English	German
general nurse (RGN)	A-Pfleger	healing	Genesung, Heilung, geistiges Heilen
generate (to)	erzeugen, verursachen, zeugen	health care	Gesundheitsfürsorge
germ	Krankheitserreger, Keim	health status	Gesundheitszustand
		health visitor	Pfleger, der Hausbesuche macht
get-well card	Grußkarte		
gland	Drüse	hearsay	Gerüchte
glossitis	Zungenentzündung	heartache	Kummer
glove	Handschuh	heartbeat	Herzschlag
goal	Ziel	heart failure	Herzversagen
goitre	Kropf	heel	Ferse
goose flesh	Gänsehaut	heel protector	Fersenschutz
gossip	Klatsch	height	Höhe
gown	Nachthemd, OP-Schürze	Heimlich manoeuvre	Heimlich-Griff
		hepatotoxicity	Leberschädlichkeit
GP (general practitioner)	Allgemeinmediziner	herbalism	Naturheilkunde
		hereditary disease	Erbkrankheit
grain	Korn, Gran	highlight (to)	betonen, hervorheben
granule	Körnchen, Granulum	hip	Hüfte
graphic	anschaulich, graphisch	Hodgkin's disease	Hodgkin-Krankheit
graphic chart	Graphik, Kurve	holistic nursing	ganzheitliche Krankenpflege
grasp (to)	ergreifen, verstehen		
greasy	fettig	home help	Haushaltshilfe
grief	Trauer	homeopathy	Homöopathie
groin	Leistengegend	honesty	Ehrlichkeit, Anständigkeit
gross national product	Bruttosozialprodukt		
guard	Schutz	hook (to)	festhaken
guess (to)	raten, vermuten	housekeeping department	Hauswirtschaftlicher Dienst
guidelines	Richtlinien		
gum	Zahnfleisch	houseman	Medizinalassistent
guts	Eingeweide	house officer	Assistenzarzt
		human response pattern	menschliche Verhaltensmuster
habit	Gewohnheit, Sucht		
haematology	Hämatologie	humerus	Oberarmknochen
haemoglobin	Hämoglobin	hydrogen peroxide	Wasserstoffperoxid
haemophilia	Hämophilie	hypertension	Bluthochdruck
haemorrhage	Blutung, Hämorrhagie	hypertrophy	Hypertrophie
hair follicle	Haarfollikel	hypnotherapy	Hypnotherapie
handgrip	Handgriff	hypothermia	Unterkühlung
hand out (to)	austeilen	hypoxia	Sauerstoffmangel
hand over (to)	weitergeben, übergeben, abgeben		
		IC nurse	Pfleger in der Intensivpflege
hanky	Taschentuch		
happen (to)	passieren	ignorance	Unwissenheit
hard	schwierig, hart	ignore (to)	ignorieren, übersehen
harm	Verletzung, Schaden	ilium	Darmbein
harmless	harmlos, ungefährlich	ill-founded	unbegründet
head (to)	an der Spitze stehen, anführen	illiteracy	Analphabetismus
		illness	Krankheit
headache	Kopfschmerz		

English	German	English	German
imaging (to)	sich vorstellen, vermu-ten	inspection	Inspektion, Untersu-chung
immediately	sofort, unverzüglich	inspiration	Einatmung, Eingebung
immune system	Immunsystem	instep	Rist
immunization	Immunisierung	instrumental (to be)	beitragen zu, behilflich sein, förderlich sein
impairment	Beeinträchtigung, Schwächung	insurance	Versicherung
impetigo	Grindflechte	insure (to)	versichern
implementation	Durchführung	integrate (to)	eingliedern, integrie-ren
implication	Auswirkung		
improper	unpassend	intention	Absicht, Vorhaben, Wundheilung
improve (to)	fördern, verbessern		
improvement	Verbesserung	interact (to)	interagieren, wechsel-wirken
impulse	Impuls		
inability	Unvermögen, Unfähig-keit	interpersonal	zwischenmenschlich
		interpolation	Einschaltung, Einfü-gung
inadequate	unzulänglich, unange-messen		
		interpretation	Deutung, Auswertung
inadvertently	versehentlich	interrupt (to)	unterbrechen
inappropriate	unpassend, unange-bracht	intervention	Eingreifen, Interventi-on, Maßnahme
inch	Inch	intestines	Eingeweide, Därme
incision	Schnittwunde, Schnitt	intolerable	unerträglich
include (to)	einschließen, enthal-ten	introduce (to)	einführen
		investigate (to)	untersuchen, erfor-schen
increase	Zunahme		
incubation period	Inkubationszeit	in vitro fertilization	In-vitro-Befruchtung
incubator	Inkubator, Brutkasten	involution	Rückbildung
independance	Unabhängigkeit	involve (to)	verwickeln, beteiligen
index finger	Zeigefinger	iodine	Jod
indicate (to)	anzeigen, hinweisen, erfordern	irregularities	Unregelmäßigkeiten, Abweichungen
indication	Hinweis, Heilanzeige	irresponsible	unverantwortlich
indifferent	gleichgültig	irreversible	unumkehrbar
industrial disease	Berufskrankheit	irritate (to)	reizen, ärgern
infertility	Unfruchtbarkeit	ischium	Sitzbein
inflammation	Entzündung	isolette	Inkubator (USA)
inflate (to)	aufblasen		
influence (to)	beeinflussen	jaundice	Gelbsucht
ingest (to)	aufnehmen, zu sich nehmen	jaw	Kiefer
		jaw bone	Kieferknochen
inhalation	Einatmung	jejunum	Leerdarm
initiate (to)	beginnen, einleiten	join (to)	verbinden, sich verei-nigen
injured	verletzt		
injurious	schädlich	joint	Gelenk
injury	Verletzung	judge	Richter
insert (to)	einführen, einstecken	judgement	Urteil
insertion	Ansatz, Einfügung	Justice	Richter
insist (to)	bestehen (auf)		
insomnia	Schlaflosigkeit	key word	Schlüsselbegriff

English	German	English	German
kidney	Niere	lock (to)	abschließen, zuschließen
kidney tray	Nierenschale		
kiss of life	Mund-zu-Mund-Beatmung	loin	Lende
		long term	Langzeit-
knee	Knie	look after (to)	versorgen
kwashiorkor	Kwashiorkor	loose weight (to)	abnehmen
		loss	Verlust
laboratory test	Labortest	loss (to be at)	sich keinen Rat wissen
labour	Wehen	loss of appetite	Appetitlosigkeit
labour (to)	in den Wehen liegen	lower case	Kleinbuchstaben
laboured	mühsam, schwerfällig	lower extremity	untere Extremität
lactation	Milchsekretion	lozenge	Tablette, Pastille
language barrier	Sprachbarriere	LPN	(in etwa Krankenpfleger)
large intestine	Dickdarm		
larynx	Kehlkopf	luxate (to)	verrenken
last (to)	andauern	LVF	linke Ventrikelinsuffizienz
last rites	Sterbesakramente		
lateral	seitlich	LVN	(in etwa Krankenpfleger)
lateral malleolus	Außenknöchel		
lateral position	Seitenlage		
laudatory	lobend	main	Haupt-
launch (to)	einführen, gründen	maintain (to)	aufrechterhalten, warten
law	Gesetz		
lead the field (to)	das Feld anführen	maintenance department	Wartungsabteilung
leadership	Führung, Leitung		
leakage	Leck	majority	Mehrheit
legislation	Gesetzgebung	make up (to)	ausdenken
lend (to)	ausleihen	malignant	bösartig
leprosy	Lepra	malnutrition	Unterernährung
lessening	Nachlassen	manipulation	Manipulation
level	Niveau	mandible	Unterkiefer
licensed	mit Erlaubnis	manual	manuell, Handbuch
lie (to)	liegen	marasmus	Verfall, Kräfteschwund
ligament	Band, Ligamentum	marble	Marmor, Murmel
limb	Gliedmaße, Extremität	mark	Mal, Fleck, Narbe
linctus	Linctus	maternity	Mutterschaft, Entbindungsstation
line (to)	auskleiden, abfüttern, überziehen		
		matter	Materie, Stoff
linen	Bettwäsche, Leinen	maxilla	Oberkiefer
liniment	Einreibmittel	means	Mittel
link with (to)	verbinden mit	measles	Masern
lint	Verbandmull	measure (to)	messen
liquid	flüssig, Flüssigkeit	measurement	Messung, Maß
list (to)	auflisten, inventarisieren	medial	medial, Mittel-
		medial malleolus	Innenknöchel
listen in on (to)	abhören, mithören	medical examination	ärztliche Untersuchung
literally	wörtlich		
little finger	kleiner Finger	medical scientist	Laborant
little toe	kleiner Zeh	meet (to)	treffen
lochia	Wochenfluss	meet with (to)	erfüllen

English	German	English	German
meeting	Versammlung	nasal cannula	Nasensonde
membrane	Membrane	nasogastric tube (NG)	Nasensonde
mental clinic	Psychiatrische Einrichtung	nausea	Übelkeit
		necessary	nötig
mental deterioration	geistiger Verfall	necessarily	notwendigerweise, unbedingt
mental disorder	Geistesstörung		
mental nurse (RMN)	B-Pfleger	neck	Hals
mentally-handicapped nurse (RNMH)	Z-Pfleger	need (to)	benötigen, brauchen
		need	Notwendigkeit, Bedürfnis
mention (to)	erwähnen		
metabolic disorder	Stoffwechselstörung	nerve	Nerv
metabolism	Stoffwechsel	neuritis	Nervenentzündung
metabolize (to)	verstoffwechseln, umwandeln	neurology	Neurologie
		neurosurgery	Neurochirurgie
metacarpals	Mittelhandknochen	nevertheless	trotzdem
metatarsals	Mittelfußknochen	newborn	Neugeborenes
micturition	Harnlassen, Urinieren	night shift	Nachtdienst
middle finger	Mittelfinger	nitrogen	Stickstoff
midnight	Mitternacht	nitrogenous	stickstoffhaltig
midwife	Hebamme	noisy	laut
minute particle	Kleinteil	non participant observation	nichtteilnehmende Beobachtung
miscarriage	Fehlgeburt		
misshapen	entstellt	nostril	Nasenloch
mixture	Gemisch, Mischung	NPO	nüchtern (Nahrung)
moist	feucht	noteworthy	bemerkenswert, beachtenswert
monitor (to)	kontrollieren, überwachen		
		notice (to)	bemerken
most commonly	meistverwendet	nourishment	Nahrung
motherhood	Mutterschaft	nursery	Kinderzimmer, Kindertageshort
mould	Schimmel, Abdruck, Guss		
		nursing care	Krankenpflege
mournful	traurig, jämmerlich	nursing mother	stillende Mutter, Pflegemutter
move bowels (to)	abführen		
movement	Bewegung	nursing officer	Leiter des Pflegedienstes
MRI (magnet resonance imaging)	NMR-Tomographie		
		nursing plan	Pflegeplan
mucous membranes	Schleimhäute	nutrients	Nährstoffe
mucus secretion	Schleimabsonderung		
multiple myeloma	Kahler-Krankheit	object (to)	dagegen sein, protestieren
multiply (to)	vervielfältigen		
mumps	Mumps	objective	objektiv, sachlich, Ziel
muscle	Muskel	observation	Beobachtung
muscle fibre	Muskelfaser	obstetric department	Geburtshilfliche Abteilung
muscular waist	Muskelatrophie		
mushroom	Pilz	obstetric nurse	Geburtshelfer
		obstruction	Verstopfung, Verschluss
NA (AN)	(in etwa Pflegehilfe)		
nail brush	Nagelbürste	obtain (to)	erhalten, erzielen
nape of the neck	Nacken	obvious	deutlich, offensichtlich
narrow	schmal, eng	occasional	gelegentlich

English	German	English	German
occipital bone	Hinterhauptsbein	pantyhose	Strumpfhose (USA)
occupational disease	Berufskrankheit	paralysis	Lähmung
occupational health nurse	betriebliche Pfleger	parasitic	parasitisch, parasitär
		parasuicide	Selbstmordversuch
occupational therapy	Beschäftigungstherapie	parietal	Scheitelbein
		partial	teilweise
occur (to)	geschehen, vorkommen, einfallen	particular	besonders, eigen
		particularly	insbesondere
oedema	Ödem	pass away (to)	sterben
oesophagus	Speiseröhre	pass urine (to)	urinieren
offend (to)	kränken, beleidigen, verstoßen (gegen)	patella	Kniescheibe
		pathology	Pathologie
often	oft	patient care unit	Patienten-Pflegeabteilung
ointment	Salbe		
olecranon process	Ellenbogenfortsatz	pattern	Muster, Schema
omit (to)	unterlassen, auslassen	PE	Lungenembolie
oncology	Onkologie	pelvic girdle	Beckengürtel
oocyte	Eizelle	pelvis	Becken
oophorectomy	Oophorektomie	peptic ulcer	peptisches Ulcus
operating theatre	OP	perambulatur (pram)	Kinderwagen
opportunity	Gelegenheit	percussion	Perkussion
oral report	mündlicher Bericht	perform (to)	ausführen, vornehmen
ordeal	Tortur, Qual	perineum	Perineum, Damm
orthopaedics	Orthopädie	permit (to)	zugestehen, erlauben
osteopathy	Osteopathie	perspiration	Transpiration
otitis media	Mittelohrentzündung	pertussis	Keuchhusten
outcome	Ergebnis	pervade (to)	sich auswirken
outlaw (to)	verbieten, ächten	phalanges	Fingerglied, Zehenglied
outlet	Öffnung, Austritt, Ventil		
		pharmacy	Apotheke
out-patient	Poliklinik, Ambulanz	phenylketonuria	Phenylketonurie
overall	gesamt, allgemein	phlegm	Schleim
over-bed table	Nachttisch mit Klappvorrichtung	physical examination	körperliche Untersuchung
overcrowded	überfüllt	physician	Arzt
overdose	Überdosis	physics	Physik
overlook (to)	überblicken, übersehen, hinwegsehen	physiotherapist	Krankengymnast
		physiotherapy	Physiotherapie
overstretch (to)	überdehnen	piles	Hämorrhoiden
oxidize (to)	oxidieren	pillow	Kissen
oxygen	Sauerstoff	pinch (to)	kneifen, quälen
oxygenation	Oxygenisation, Sauerstoffanreicherung	pint	Pint (Hohlmaß)
		plague	Pest, Seuche
		plaster (of Paris)	Gips
pad	Polster, Kompresse	plastic surgery	Plastische Chirurgie
paediatric ward	Kinderstation	poison	Gift
pale	bleich, blass	poisonous	giftig
pallid	bleich, blass	poll	Meinungsumfrage
pallor	Bleichheit, Blässe	poll (to)	untersuchen
panties	Slip	pollution	Verschmutzung

English	German	English	German
pool	Schwimmbecken	probe	Sonde
poor eyesight	schwache Augen	proceed (to)	fortsetzen, fortfahren
poor hearing	schlechte Ohren	progress	Fortschritt, Fortgang
popliteal space	Kniekehle	progress (to)	entwickeln, fortschrei-
population	Bevölkerung		ten
position	Haltung, Position	progressive	zunehmend, fort-
post-holder	Stelleninhaber		schreitend
potassium	Kaliumpermanganat	prolonged period	längerer Zeitraum
permanganate		promptly	unmittelbar
potential	potentiell	properly	richtig, anständig
practice	Praxis, Erfahrung	prophylactic	prophylaktisch
practice nurse	medizinischer Assis-	prostate gland	Prostata, Vorsteher-
	tent		drüse
praise	Lob	protective	beschützend
predictable	vorhersehbar	protein	Eiweiß
predominant	vorherrschend	protozoa	Protozoen
prefer (to)	vorziehen, lieber mö-	prove (to)	beweisen
	gen	provide (to)	bereitstellen, zur Ver-
preference	Vorzug		fügung stellen
pregnant	schwanger	psychotherapy	Psychotherapie
premature	Frühgeborenes, früh-	pubis	Schambein
	reif, vorzeitig	public health	öffentliche Gesundheit
preparation	Vorbereitung, Ausbil-	public place	öffentlicher Platz
	dung	puff adder	Puffotter
prepare (to)	vorbereiten	pulse	Puls, Pulsschlag
prepared	vorbereitet	punishment	Strafe
preposition	Präposition	purpose	Zweck, Absicht
prescribe (to)	vorschreiben, ver-	push (to)	stoßen, schieben,
	schreiben, verord-		drücken
	nen	pylorus	Magenpförtner
prescription	Rezept		
present	anwesend, Gegenwart	q2h	alle 2 Stunden
presented	überreicht, vorgelegt	qualification	Qualifikation, Zeugnis,
preserve (to)	bewahren, erhalten,		Abschluss
	konservieren	quantity	Menge
press (to)	pressen	quiet	ruhig, still
pressure	Druck	quit (to)	verlassen, kündigen
pressure area	Druckstelle	quote (to)	zitieren, anführen
pressure ulcer	Druckgeschwür, Deku-		
	bitus	rabies	Tollwut
presumption	Annahme, Vermutung	radial	Radius, Radial-
pretend (to)	vorgeben	radiation	Strahlung
pretty	hübsch	radioactive	radioaktiv
prevent (to)	vermeiden, verhüten	radiology	Röntgen
preventative teaching	präventive Ausbildung	radius	Radius, Speiche, Wir-
previous	vorausgehend		kungsbereich
primarily	hauptsächlich	rails	Bettgitter
principal	hauptsächlich, Haupt-	raise (to)	heben, hochziehen,
PRN	wie gewünscht		großziehen
probably	wahrscheinlich	rale (crepitation)	Rasseln

English	German	English	German
randomly	zufällig, willkürlich	remedial	heilend, Heil-
rapid(ly)	schnell	remission	vorübergehende Bes-
rare	selten		serung
rash	Ausschlag	remove (to)	entfernen
rate	Geschwindigkeit	renal failure	Niereninsuffizienz
ratio	Verhältnis, Quotient	renal unit	Dialyseabteilung
rationale	logische Grundlage, Grundprinzip	repair (to)	reparieren
		repeatedly	wiederholt
readmit (to)	wiederaufnehmen, wiedereinweisen	replication	Replikation, Verdoppe-lung
realignment	Wiederausrichtung	reproduce (to)	fortpflanzen, züchten
reassure (to)	beruhigen, beteuern	reproductive system	Fortpflanzungsorgane
receive (to)	erhalten	request (to)	bitten, ersuchen
recipient	Empfänger	require (to)	benötigen, brauchen, erfordern
recognize (to)	erkennen, wiederer-kennen	requirement	Bedarf, Anspruch, Er-fordernis
recommendation	Empfehlung		
record (to)	aufnehmen, aufzeich-nen, dokumentie-ren	resource	Mittel, Quelle, Res-sourcen
		with respect to	in Bezug auf, bezüg-lich
records	Dokumente, Akten		
record sheet	Formular	respiration	Atmung
recovery	Genesung	respiratory	Atmung betreffend
recovery position	stabile Seitenlage	respond (to)	antworten, reagieren, ansprechen
rectum	Rektum, Enddarm		
reduce (to)	reduzieren, verringern	responsibility	Verantwortung
refer to (to)	erwähnen, sich bezie-hen auf	responsible	verantwortlich
		responsive	antwortend, anspre-chend, empfänglich
reference	Bemerkung, Bezug		
reflexology	Reflexzonentherapie	responsiveness	Reaktionsvermögen, Empfänglichkeit
refuse (to)	ablehnen, zurückwei-sen		
		restore (to)	wiederherstellen
regain consciousness (to)	zu Bewusstsein kom-men, Bewusstsein wiedererlangen	restrict (to)	einschränken
		resuscitation	Reanimation, Wieder-belebung
regarding	bezüglich, in Bezug auf	retain (to)	behalten, zurückhal-ten
register (to)	einschreiben, regis-trieren	retirement	Pensionierung, Ruhe-stand
reiterate (to)	wiederholen	retraining of bladder	Blasentest
reject (to)	abstoßen, ablehnen, zurückweisen	retrospective	rückblickend, Retro-spektive
relapse	Rückfall	return (to)	zurückkommen
relationship	Beziehung	reversal	Umkehrung, Um-schlag
release (to)	freigeben, befreien		
relief	Erleichterung, Hilfe	review (to)	zurückblicken, über-prüfen
relief (to)	erleichtern, lindern		
rely on (to)	angewiesen auf, sich verlassen auf	reward (to)	belohnen
		rickets	Rachitis
remain to be seen	zu beweisen bleiben	rid (to)	befreien

English	German	English	German
rigorous	strikt, gründlich	severe	ernsthaft
ring finger	Ringfinger	severity	Strenge, Ernst, Stärke
rise (to)	steigen, aufstehen	sexual advances	sexuelle Belästigung
rock (to)	schaukeln, wiegen	shaped	geformt
root	Wurzel	share (to)	teilen
rope	Tau, Seil, Strang, Strick	sheepskin	Schafsfell
roster	Dienstplan	sheet	Laken
rota	Dienstplan	shifts (to work in)	Schichtdienst (arbeiten)
rotate (to)	rotieren, sich abwechseln	shine (to)	scheinen
rub (to)	reiben	shirt	Oberhemd, Bluse
rule	Regel, Richtlinie	shiver (to)	zittern
ruling	leitend, vorherrschend	SHO	1. Promotion nach Approbation des Arztes
runny	dünn, flüssig		
rupture (to)	brechen, zerreißen		
		shoehorn	Schuhlöffel
sack (to)	entlassen	shortness of breath	Kurzatmigkeit
sacrum	Kreuzbein	shoulder	Schulter
safe environment	sichere Umgebung	shoulder blade	Schulterblatt
safety pin	Sicherheitsnadel	shower	Dusche
sample	Muster	shrink (to)	eingehen, kleiner werden
scales	Waage		
scapula	Schulterblatt	sibling	Bruder, Schwester
scheme	Schema	sick (to be)	sich übergeben
schistosomiasis	Bilharziose	sick children's nurse (RSCN)	Pfleger für Kinderpflege
school nurse	Schulkrankenpfleger		
scientific	wissenschaftlich	sickle cell anaemia	Sichelzellenanämie
scissors	Schere	side effect	Nebenwirkung
scream (to)	schreien, aufschreien	sight	Sehvermögen
screening	Durchleuchtung	sign and symptom	Zeichen und Symptom
scurvy	Skorbut	signal cord	Klingelknopf
SDAT	Alzheimer	significant	wichtig, bedeutend
second opinion	zusätzliche Beratung	silicosis	Steinstaublunge
second (2nd) toe	zweiter Zeh	similarity	Ähnlichkeit, Gleichartigkeit
secrete (to)	absondern		
secretion	Absonderung, Sekretion	simile	Vergleich
		Sims's position	linke Seitenlage mit hochgezogenem rechten Knie
secure a hold (to)	Einfluss nehmen		
sedative	Beruhigungsmittel		
seize (to)	packen, ergreifen	sinoatrial node	Sinusknoten
seizure	plötzlicher Anfall	sister	Schwester, Stationsschwester
select (to)	auswählen		
self-esteem	Selbstachtung	skill	Fertigkeit
self-help skills	Selbsthilfe	skin colour	Hautfarbe
sensitive	sensibel, empfindlich	skin disorder	Hautkrankheit
separate (to)	scheiden, trennen	skin folds	Hautfalten
separated by	getrennt durch	skull	Schädel
separately	separat	slacks	kurze Hosen (USA)
settle down (to)	beruhigen, ruhiger werden	slap	Schlag, Klaps
		sleeve	Ärmel

English	German	English	German
sling	Armschlinge	statement	Aussage
slip (to)	schieben, gleiten rutschen	status	Zustand
		status quo	unveränderter Zustand
slippers	Pantoffeln		
sliver	Splitter	statute	Gesetz, Satzung
slurred speech	verwaschene Sprache	sternum	Brustbein
small intestine	Dünndarm	stiffness	Steifheit
smart	schick, gewitzt, rasch	sitpulate (to)	verlangen, festsetzen, vorschreiben
smooth	glatt		
snake bite	Schlangenbiss	stitch	Stich, Naht
snap (to)	schnippen, schnalzen, brechen	stitch (to)	nähen
		stockinette	Trikotstrumpf, Schlauchbinde
snoring	Schnarchen		
soaked	durchnässt, eingeweicht	stomach	Magen
		stools	Stuhlgang
sober	nüchtern (Alkohol)	storm (to)	stürmen, toben
social security	soziale Sicherheit	strap	Riemen, Gurt, Band
social services	Sozialarbeit	straight	gerade
soft tissues	weiche Tücher	straw	Röhrchen
soiled	schmutzig, verschmutzt	strength	Kraft, Stärke
		stretch (to)	strecken, dehnen, spannen
solid waste	feste Abfallstoffe		
solution	Lösung	stretcher	Krankenbahre
solve (to)	lösen	stroke	Schlaganfall
sore	entzündet, wund	subnormal	Minderbegabter, unterdurchschnittlich
sound asleep (to be)	tief schlafen		
source	Quelle	subsequent	nachfolgend
species	Gattung, Art	substance	Stoff, Substanz
specific	spezifisch, kennzeichnend	substract (to)	abziehen
		suction	Saugen, Saugwirkung, Sog
specimen	(Gewebs-, Blut-, Urin-) Probe		
		sufferer	Leidender, -kranker
spectacles (specs)	Brille	suffer from (to)	leiden an
speech	Sprechvermögen	suffocate (to)	ersticken, würgen
speech therapy	Logopädie	suggest (to)	vorschlagen, anregen, andeuten
sphygmomanometer	Blutdruckmessgerät		
spinal cord	Rückenmark	suicide	Selbstmord
spine	Dorn, Fortsatz, Stachel	suit (to)	passen, bekommen (Essen)
spit (to)	spucken		
spleen	Milz	suitable	geeignet, passend
splinter	Splitter	supplementary	ergänzend, zusätzlich
spot	Fleck, Pustel, Hautmal		
sprain (to)	verstauchen, dehnen, zerren	supply (to)	sorgen für, liefern
		support	Unterstützung
spread	Verbreitung, Umfang, Abweichung	support (to)	unterstützen
		suppository	Zäpfchen
stabbing pain	stechender Schmerz	suppress (to)	unterdrücken
stability	Stabilität	surface	Oberfläche, Fläche
staff	Personal	surgeon	Chirurg
standardise	vereinheitlichen	surgery	Operation, Chirurgie

English	German	English	German
run surgery (to)	Sprechstunde abhalten	threat	Drohung, Bedrohung, Gefahr
surgery hours	Sprechstunde	throat	Kehle, Rachen, Hals
surprising(ly)	überraschend	throbbing	Klopfen, Pochen
surrogacy	Leihmutterschaft	thrush	Mundsoor
surround (to)	umgeben	thrust	Stoß, Druckkraft
survey	Überblick, Übersicht, Reihenuntersuchung	thumb	Daumen
		thyroid gland	Schilddrüse
		thyroxine	Thyroxin
survive (to)	überleben	tibia	Tibia, Schienbein
suspicious	argwöhnisch, misstrauisch	TID	3x täglich
		tie off (to)	abbinden
sustain (to)	aushalten, erhalten, aufrechterhalten	tighten (to)	spannen, festziehen, straffen
swallow (to)	schlucken	tights	Strumpfhosen
swelling	Schwellung	tilt (to)	kippen, neigen, schräg stellen
swollen	angeschwollen		
symmetry	Symmetrie	time span	Zeitspanne, Zeitumfang
symphysis pubis	Schambeinknorpelfuge		
		tiredness	Müdigkeit, Übermüdung
snythetic	Kunststoff, synthetisch		
syringe	Spritze	toe	Zeh
systemic	Gesamtorganismus betreffend	toiletries	Toilettenartikel
		tombstone	Grabstein
systolic pressure	systolischer Druck	tonsillectomy	Tonsillenentfernung
		tool	Werkzeug
tail	Schwanz	tooth	Zahn
tail (to)	beschatten, folgen	tourniquet	Aderpresse
tap (to)	anzapfen, klopfen	towards	in Richtung, auf ... zu, gegenüber
tarsal	Fußwurzel(-knochen)		
task	Aufgabe	toxic	giftig
tea	Tee, Abendessen	TPN	vollständige parenterale Ernährung
temporary	vorübergehend, befristet		
		TPR values	TPR-Werte
tempting	verführerisch, verlockend	trachea	Luftröhre
		traction	Traktion, Zug, Ziehen
tend towards (to)	geneigt sein zu	train (to)	ausbilden, schulen
tendon	Sehne	transfer	Transfer, Übertragung, Verlegung
tension	Spannung, Anspannung		
		transfusion	Transfusion
theatre nurse	OP-Pfleger	transmit (to)	übertragen, vererben, weiterleiten
thesis	These, Behauptung, Doktorarbeit		
		transperitoneal	durch die Bauchdecke
thick	dick, überflüssig, heiser	transverse	quer, transversal
		trapeze	Trapez
thicken (to)	verdicken, eindicken, trüben	trauma	Trauma
		treat (to)	behandeln
thigh	Oberschenkel	treatment	Behandlung
third (3rd) toe	dritter Zeh	treatment room	Behandlungszimmer
thorough(ly)	tiefgehend, gründlich	trial	Versuch, Probe, Test

English	German	English	German
trolley	Handwagen, Teewagen	use	Verwendung, Benutzung, Einnahme
trunk	Rumpf	usually	üblicherweise, gewöhnlich
trusting	vertrauensvoll, gutgläubig	uterus	Gebärmutter
truth	Wahrheit		
tube-feeding	Ernährung mit Sonde	vaccine	Impfstoff
turn (to)	umdrehen, drehen, wenden	vacuum extraction	Vakuumextraktion
		vaginal examination	Vaginaluntersuchung
tweezers	Pinzette	value (to be of)	wichtig sein, wertvoll sein
twins	Zwillinge		
typhoid fever	Typhus	value judgement	Werturteil
		variance	Unterschied
ulcer	Ulkus, Geschwür	at variance with (to be)	anderer Meinung sein
ulna	Elle		
umbilical cord	Nabelschnur	varicectomy	Entfernen der Krampfadern
unanimously	einstimmig		
uncertainty	Unsicherheit	vary (to)	abwechseln, wechseln
undergo surgery (to)	sich einer Operation unterziehen	vascular surgery	Gefäßchirurgie
		vector	Träger, Vektor
underlie (to)	zugrunde liegen	vegetable life	pflanzlicher Organismus
underpants	Unterhose (UK)		
undershirt	Unterhemd (USA)	venom	Gift
underwear	Unterwäsche	vernix caseosa	Vernix caseosa
undress (to)	auskleiden, ausziehen	vertebra	Wirbel
unfair	ungerecht, unlauter	vertebral column	Wirbelsäule
unfavourable	ungünstig, widrig	vessel	Gefäß, Ader
unfold (to)	entwickeln, entfalten, ausbreiten	vest	Unterhemd (UK), Weste (USA)
uniform	einheitlich, gleichmäßig, eintönig	vicious	gehässig, gemein, boshaft, mangelhaft
unnecessary	unnötig		
unusual(ly)	ungewöhnlich, außergewöhnlich	victim	Opfer
		violate (to)	verstoßen gegen, vergewaltigen
update (to)	auf den neuesten Stand bringen	visible	sichtbar, deutlich
uplifting	erhebend, erbaulich	vision	Sehkraft, Halluzination
upper body	Oberkörper	vital signs	primäre Lebenszeichen
upper end	Oberseite		
upper extremity	Arm	vomit (to)	sich erbrechen
upset	bestürzt, ärgerlich, gekränkt		
		wages	Lohn
urge (to)	drängen, eindringlich bitten	waist	Taille
		waiting room	Wartezimmer
urgent laboratory	Notfalllabor	walker	Laufstuhl
urinal	Bettflasche	wall	Wand
urination	Urinieren	ward	Station
urine test	Urinuntersuchung	wash-out	Ausspülung, Auswaschung
urology	Urologie		
		waste	Abfall

English	German	English	German
watch (to)	schauen, überwachen, beobachten	wipe (to)	wischen, aufwischen
		wit	Verstand, Geist, Witz
water-birth	Wassergeburt	witty	witzig, geistreich
weakness	Schwäche	worry (to)	sich Sorgen machen
wealthy	reich	wound disruption	Aufbrechen einer Wunde
wedge (to)	einzwängen, verklemmen		
		wrap (to)	einpacken, einwickeln
well-dressed	gut gekleidet	wrinkled	zerknittert, faltig
wellness	Wohlbefinden, Gesundsein	wrist	Handwurzel
well-off	reich, begütert	xerophthalmia	Xerophthalmie
wet (to)	befeuchten, nass machen	xiphoid process	Schwertfortsatz
		X-ray	Röntgenaufnahme
wheat germ	Weizenkeim	X-ray department	Röntgenabteilung
whipworm	Peitschenwurm		
whites of the eyes	Weiß der Augen	yeast	Hefe, Sprosspilz
whooping cough	Keuchhusten	yellowish	gelblich
willingness	Bereitwilligkeit		
windpipe	Luftröhre	zip	Zischen, Reißverschluss
wind up (to)	aufziehen (Uhr), enden		
		zygomatic bone	Jochbein

Vocabulary: German-English

Für alle Berufe gilt sowohl die männliche als auch die weibliche Form. Die Übersetzung der Wörter bezieht sich in den meisten Fällen auf den Kontext dieses Buches.

German	English	German	English
A-Pfleger	general nurse (RGN)	Aderpresse	tourniquet
abbinden	to tie off	Adoption	adoption
Abendessen	tea	Ähnlichkeit	similarity
Abfall	waste	Akkupunktur	acupuncture
abfällig	derogatory	Akromion	acromion
abfällige Bemerkung	aspersion	Akronym	acronym
Abfallprodukt	byproduct	Akten	records
abführen	to move bowels	aktuell	current
abfüttern (mit Stoff)	to line	akut	acute
abgeben	to hand over	alle 2 Stunden	q2h
abhalten	to discourage	allgemein	common(ly), overall
abhängig sein von	to depend on	Allgemeinheit	community
Abhören	auscultation	Allgemeinmediziner	general practitioner (GP)
abkühlen	to chill		
Abkürzung	abbreviation	Altenpflege	care of the elderly
ablassen (Luft)	to deflate	ältere	elderly
ablehnen	to refuse, to reject	ältlich	elderly
Ablehnung	denial	Alzheimer	SDAT
ableiten (von)	to derive	ambulant	ambulant
Abnahme (Wert)	decrease	Ambulanz	out-patient
abnehmen (Gewicht)	to lose weight	Analphabetismus	illiteracy
abraten	to discourage	Anamnese	case history
Abruck	mould	andauern	to last
abschätzig	derogatory	anderer Meinung sein	to be at variance with
abscheiden	to excrete	Änderung	amendment
abschließen	to lock	andeuten	to suggest
Abschluss (Schule)	degree, qualification	Anfall	fit
Absicht	intention, purpose, aim	anführen	to head (leiten), to quote (zitieren)
absichtlich	deliberate	angeboren	congenital
absondern	to secrete	angeschwollen	swollen
Absonderung	discharge, secretion	angewiesen auf	to rely on
abstoßen	to reject	Angst	anxiety, fear
Abszess	abscess	ängstlich	frightened
abwechseln	to vary, ro rotate	anheften	to stick
abwechselnd	alternately	ankleben	to stick
Abweichung	abnormality, spread, irregularity	Annäherung	approach
		Annahme	presumption
abwickeln	to unwind	Anordnung	arrangement
abziehen	to substract	anregen	to suggest
Achsel	armpit, axilla	Ansatz	approach, insertion
ächten	to outlaw	anschaulich	graphic
Ader	vessel	anschließen	to connect

German	English	German	English
ansehnlich	considerable	Aufbrechen einer Wunde	wound disruption
Anspannung	tension		
ansprechen	to address, to respond (Medikament)	Aufgabe	task
		aufgrund	due to
ansprechend	responsive	Aufklärung	enlightenment
Anspruch	requirement	auflisten	to list
anständig	properly	Aufmerksamkeit	attention
Anständigkeit	honesty	Aufnahme	admission
ansteigen	to rise	Aufnahme Urinunter-	ASU
anstellen	to employ	suchung	
Antiazidum	antacid	aufnehmen	to ingest (Nahrung
antiseptisch	antiseptic		etc.), to record
antworten	to respond		(Musik), to admit
antwortend	responsive		(ins Krankenhaus)
anwenden	to employ	aufrechterhalten	to maintain, to sustain
Anwendung	application	Aufreißen einer Wun-	wound disruption
anwesend sein	to be present, to at-	de	
	tend	aufschreien	to scream
anzapfen	to tap	aufstehen	to rise
anzeigen	to indicate	aufstellen (Plan)	to draw up
anziehen	to dress	in Auftrag geben	to commission
anzünden	to light	aufwachen	to awake
Apathie	apathy	aufwischen	to wipe
Apotheke	pharmacy	aufzeichnen	to record
Appetitlosigkeit	loss of appetite	aufziehen	to draw up, to wind up
ärgerlich	upset	Aufzug	elevator
ärgern	to irritate	Ausatmung	exhalation, expiration
argwöhnisch	suspicious	ausbilden	to train
Arm	upper extremity,	Ausbildung	preparation
	arm	Ausbildung betreffend	educational
Ärmel	sleeve	Ausbildungserfahrung	educational experi-
Ärmelloch	arm hole		ence
Armschlinge	sling	ausbreiten	to spread, to unfold
Arrhythmie	arrhythmia	ausdehnen	to dilate, to expand
Art	character, species	Ausdehnung	dilatation (UK),
Arterien betreffend	arterial		dilation (USA)
Arzneimittelvergabe	drug round	ausdenken	to make up
Arzt	physician	Ausdruck	expression
ärztliche Untersu-	medical examination	ausdrücken	to express
chung		ausführen	to carry out, to per-
Assistenzarzt	house officer		form
Atem	breath	Ausgaben	expenditures
Atemdepression	respiratory depression	ausgeben	to spend
Ätiologie	etiology	aushalten	to sustain
Atmung	respiration	aushusten	to expectorate
Atmung betreffend	respiratory	auskleiden	to line (mit Stoff), to
ätzend	caustic		undress (Kleidung)
auf ... zu	towards	auslassen	to omit
Aufbau	construction	ausleihen	to lend
aufblasen	to inflate	Auspressen	expression

German	English	German	English
ausrotten	to eradicate	bedeutend	significant, important
Ausrüstung	equipment	Bedingung	condition
Aussage	statement	Bedrohung	threat
ausschaben	to erase	Bedürfnis	need
ausscheiden	to excrete	beeinflussen	to affect, to influence
Ausscheidung	discharge, elimination	Beeinträchtigung	impairment
Ausschlag	rash	beenden	to conclude, to finish
Ausschluss	exclusion	befähigen	to enable
Ausschneiden	excision	befehlen	to command
Ausschnitt	cutting	befestigen	to attach, to fasten
Außenknöchel	lateral malleolus	befeuchten	to wet
außergewöhnlich	unusual(ly)	befreien	to release, to rid
ausspülen	to flush	befristet	temporary
Ausspülung	wash-out	Befruchtung	conception
austeilen	to dispense, to hand out	Befund	findings
		beginnen	to commence, to begin, to initiate
Austreibung	expulsion		
Austritt	outlet	begütert	well-off
Austrocknung	dehydration	behalten	to keep, to retain
ausüben	to exert	behandeln	to attend, to treat
auswählen	to choose, to select	Behandlung	attendance, cure, treatment
Auswaschung	wash-out		
auswerten	to evaluate	Behandlungszimmer	treatment room, surgery
Auswertung	interpretation, evaluation		
		behaupten	to claim
sich auswirken	to pervade	Behauptung	allegation, thesis
Auswirkung	implication	behilflich sein	to be instrumental
Auszeichnung	distinction	Behinderung	disturbance
ausziehen	to undress	Beispiel	example
Autoimmunerkrankung	autoimmune desease	beißen	to bite
		beitragen	to contribute, to be instrumental
B-Pfleger	mental nurse (RMN)		
baden	to bathe	bekommen	to get, to suit (Essen)
Badezimmer	bathroom	belästigen	to bother
Band	ligament (anat.), strap (Riemen)	belauschen	to eavesdrop
		belegen	to audit
Barmherzigkeit	charity	beleidigen	to offend
Bettbahre	bedcradle	beleuchten	to light
Bauch	abdomen, belly	belohnen	to reward
Bauch betreffend	abdominal	bemerken	to notice
durch die Bauchdecke	transperitoneal	bemerkenswert	noteworthy
bauen	to build	Bemerkung	comment, reference
beachtenswert	noteworthy	benötigen	to need, to require
beanspruchen	to claim	Benutzung	use
beauftragen	to commission	beobachten	to watch
Becken	pelvis	Beobachtung	observation
Beckengürtel	pelvic girdle	beratend	consultative
Bedarf	requirement	Beratung	counselling
bedecken	to cover	bereitstellen	to provide
bedenken	to consider	Bereitwilligkeit	willingness

German	English	German	English
bersten	to burst	Beweis	evidence
berücksichtigen	to take into account, to consider	beweisen	to prove
		zu beweisen bleiben	remain to be seen
Berufskrankheit	industrial disease, occupational disease	bewerten	to evaluate
		bewundern	to admire
beruhigen	to reassure, to settle down	bewusst	deliberate
		das Bewusstsein wiedererlangen	to regain consciousness
Beruhigungsmittel	sedative		
beschädigt	damaged	zu Bewusstsein kommen	to regain consciousness
beschäftigen	to employ		
Beschäftigungstherapie	occupational therapy	Bewusstseinsstörung	disturbed consciousness
beschneiden	to circumcise	bezahlen	to pay
Beschreibung	description	sich beziehen auf	to refer to
Beschuldigung	accusation	Beziehung	relationship
beschützend	protective	Bezug	reference
Beschwerde	complaint, discomfort (körperlich)	in bezug auf	in respect of, regarding
beschweren	to complain	bezüglich	in respect of, regarding
Beseitigung	elimination		
besonders	particular	BH	bra
Besorgnis	anxiety, concern	Bikinischnitt	bikini cut
Besserung	amendment	Bilharziose	schistosomiasis
Bestätigung	confirmation	billig	cheap
Bestehen	existence	Billigkeit	equity
bestehen auf	to insist on	Bindehaut	conjunctiva
bestehen aus	to consist of	binden	to bind
bestimmen	to determine	bitten	to request
bestürzt	upset	Blase	bladder
beteiligen	to involve	blasen	to blow
Beteiligung	contribution	Blasentest	retraining of bladder
beteuern	to reassure	blass	pallid, pale
betonen	to emphasize, to highlight	Blässe	pallor
		blauer Fleck	bruise
betrachten	to consider	bleich	pallid, pale
beträchtlich	considerable	Bleichheit	pallor
betrieblicher Pfleger	occupational health nurse	den Blick erweitern	to broaden a scope
		Bluse	blouse, shirt
das Bett hüten müssen	to be confined to bed	Blutdruck	blood pressure (BP)
Bettflasche	urinal	Blutdruckmessgerät	sphygmomanometer
Bettgitter	rails	bluten	to bleed
Bettpfanne	bedpan	Bluthochdruck	hypertension
Bettwäsche	linen	Blutkrankheit	blood disorder
Bettzeug	bedclothes	Blutkreislauf	circulation
beugen	to bend	Blutprobe	blood sample
beunruhigend	disturbing	Bluttransfusion	transfusion
beurteilen	to assess	Blutung	haemorrhage
Bevölkerung	population	Blutverlust	blood loss
bewahren	to preserve	Blutzuckerspiegel	blood sugar level
Bewegung	movement	bösartig	malignant

German	English	German	English
boshaft	vicious	eine Diagnose stellen	to confirm a diagnosis
Bradykardie	bradycardia	Dialyseabteilung	renal unit
Brand	gangrene	Diaphragma	diaphragm
brauchen	to need, to require	Diarrhoe	diarrhoea
brechen	to break, to rupture, to snap	diastolischer Druck	diastolic pressure
		dick	thick
Brechschale	emesis basin	Dickdarm	colon, large intestine
Brennen	burning feeling	dickflüssig	thick
brennen	to burn	Dienstplan	roster, rota
Brille	spactacles, specs	Diskussion	debate
bringen	to bring	dispensieren	to dispense
Bronchoskopie	bronchoscopy	Doktorarbeit	thesis
Bruch	fracture	Dokumente	records
Brust	chest	dokumentieren	to record
Brustbein	sternum	Dollar	buck
Brustkorb	chest	Dorn	spine
Brutkasten	incubator	Dosierung	dosage
Bruttosozialprodukt	gross national product	Dosis	dosage
buchstabieren	to spell	Dragee	coated tablet
Bundes-	federal	drängen	to urge
		drehen	to turn
Candidose	candidosis	dreimal täglich	TID
Chemiebetrieb	chemical plant	Drogenabhängiger	drug addict
Chirurg	surgeon	Drogist	chemist
Chirurgie	surgery	Drohung	threat
chronisch-obstruktive Atemwegserkran-kung	COAD	Druck	pressure
		drücken	to push
		Druckgeschwür	pressure ulcer
circa	approximately	Druckkraft	thrust
computergesteuerte Aufzeichnung	computerized event recorder	Druckstelle	pressure area
		Drüse	gland
		dünn	runny
dagegen sein	to object	Dünndarm	small intestine
Damm	perineum	durchbrechen	to breach
Darm	bowel	Durchführung	implementation
Darmbein	ilium	Durchleuchtung	screening
Därme	intestines	durchnässt	soaked
Darmentleerung	defecation	Dusche	shower
Dauer	duration	Dyspepsie	dyspepsia
Daumen	thumb		
Daunen	fluff	ebenso	alike
Debatte	debate	effektiv	effective(ly)
Decke	blanket	Ehrlichkeit	honesty
dehnen	to sprain, to stretch	Eidotter	egg yolk
Dekubitus	pressure ulcer	eigen	particulur
delegieren	to delegate	Einatmung	inhalation, inspiration
denken	to think	eindicken	to thicken
Dermatologie	dermatology	eindringlich bitten	to urge
deutlich	obvious, visible	einfallen	to occur
Deutung	interpretation	Einfluss nehmen	to secure a hold

German	English	German	English
einfrieren	to freeze	eng	narrow
Einfügung	insertion, interpolation	entbinden	to deliver
		Entbindung	delivery
einführen	to establish, to insert, to introduce, to launch	Entbindungsstation	maternity
		entfalten	to unfold
		entfernen	to remove
eingebaut	built-in	Entfernen der Krampfadern	varicectomy
Eingebung	inspiration		
eingehen	to shrink	Entfernung	elimination, excision
eingeweicht	soaked	entgegenwirken	to counteract
Eingeweide	guts, intestines	enthalten	to contain, to include
eingliedern	to integrate	entlassen	to sack
Eingreifen	intervention	Entlassung	discharge
einheitlich	uniform	entmutigen	to discourage
in Einklang mit	corresponding	entmutigt	demoralized
einleiten	to initiate	Entscheidung	decision
Einnahme	use	Entschluss	decision
einpacken	to wrap	entsprechend	corresponding, according to
Einreibmittel	liniment		
Einschaltung	interpolation	entstehen	to arise
Einschätzung	assessment	entstellt	misshapen
einschließen	to include	entwickeln	to evolve, to develop, to progress, to unfold
einschränken	to restrict		
einschreiben	to register		
einstecken	to insert	Entwicklung	development
einstellen	to adjust	entwirren	to unwind
einstimmig	unanimously	entziehen	to deprive of
eintönig	unifrom	entzündet	sore
einverstanden sein	to approve	Entzündung	inflammation
einwickeln	to wrap	Episiotomie	episiotomy
einzwängen	to wedge	erachten	to deem
Eitergeschwür	abscess	erbauend	uplifting
Eiweiß	protein	Erbkrankheit	hereditary disease
Eizelle	oocyte	sich erbrechen	to vomit
Ekzem	eczema	Erfahrung	practice
Elixier	elixir	erfordern	to indicate, to require
Elle	ulna	Erfordernis	requirement
Ellenbogen	elbow	erforschen	to investigate, to explore
Ellenbogenfortsatz	olecranon process		
Embolie	embolism	erfüllen	to meet with
empfangen	to conceive	ergänzend	supplementary, complementary
Empfänger	recipient		
empfänglich	responsive	Ergebnis	outcome
Empfänglichkeit	responsiveness	ergreifen	to grasp, to seize
Empfängnis	conception	erhalten	to obtain, to receive, to derive, to preserve (konservieren), to sustain (aufrechterhalten)
Empfehlung	recommendation		
empfindlich	sensitive		
Enddarm	rectum		
enden	to wind up		
endogen	endogenous		

German	English	German	English
erhebend	uplifting	fallen	to fall
erhöhen	to enhance	falsch	false
erkennen	to distinguish, to recognize	faltig	wrinkled
		fangen	to catch
erklären	to account for, to explain	Faser	fibre
		aus der Fassung bringen	to upset
Erkrankung	disorder		
erlauben	to allow, to permit	fassungslos	flabbergasted
mit Erlaubnis	licensed	fegen	to sweep
erledigen	to finish	fehlerhaft	false
erleichtern	to relieve	Fehlgeburt	miscarriage
Erleichterung	ease, relief	das Feld anführen	to lead the field
Erleuchtung	enlightenment	Ferse	heel
Ermüdung	fatigue	Fersenbein	calcaneus
ernähren	to feed	Fersenschutz	heel protector
Ernährung mit Sonde	tube-feeding	Fertigkeit	ability, skill
Ernst	severity	fest	firm(ly)
ernsthaft	severe, critically	feste Abfallstoffe	solid waste
erreichen	to achieve	festhaken	to hook
erröten	to flush	sich festklammern	to cling
erscheinen	to appear	festsetzen	to stipulate
Erschöpfung	fatigue	feststellen	to determine
erschrocken	frightened	Feststellung	assessment
Erste Hilfe	accident and emergency	festziehen	to tighten
		fettig	greasy
ersticken	to choke, to suffocate	feucht	moist
ersuchen	to request	Fieber	fever
ertränken	to drown	Fieberkurve	chart
erwähnen	to refer to, to mention	Finanzabteilung	business department
erwarten	to expect	Finanzierung	funding
erwartungsvoll	expectant	finden	to find
erweitern	to dilate	Fingerglied	phalanges
Erweiterung	dilatation (UK), dilation (USA), enlargement	Fläche	surface
		mit der Flasche ernähren	to bottle-feed
Erweiterung und Ausschabung	D & C		
		Flaum	fluff
erzählen	to tell	Fleck	mark, spot
erzeugen	to generate	fliegen	to fly
erzielen	to obtain	flüchten	to flee
essen	to eat	Fluss	flow
Exaktheit	conciseness	flüssig	liquid, runny
Existenz	existence	Flüssigkeit	fluid, liquid
exogen	exogenous	Flüssigkeitsausscheidung	fluid output
Extremität	limb		
		Flüssigkeitszufuhr	fluid intake
Facharzt	consultant	föderativ	federal
Fähigkeit	ability	fokussieren	to focus
fahren	to drive, to ride	Folgen	consequences
Fairness	equity	folgern	to conclude
Fall	case	förderlich sein	to be instrumental

German	English	German	English
fordern	to call for, to demand	Gefäß	vessel
fördern	to improve	Gefäßchirurgie	vascular surgery
Formulare	record sheets	geformt	shaped
fortfahren	to proceed	gegen den Rat der Ärzte	AMA
Fortgang	progress		
fortpflanzen	to reproduce	Gegengift	antidote, antivenom
Fortpflanzungsorgane	reproductive system	gegenüber	towards
Fortsatz	spine	Gegenwart	present
fortschreiten	to progress	gehässig	vicious
fortschreitend	progressive	gehen	to go
Fortschritt	progress	Gehirn	brain
fortsetzen	to continue, to proceed	Gehorsam	compliance
		Geist	wit
Fötus	foetus, fetus	Geistesstörung	mental disorder
Fraktur	fracture	geistiges Heilen	healing
freigeben	to release	geistiger Verfall	mental deterioration
Fremdkörper	foreign body	geistreich	witty
frieren	to freeze	gekränkt	upset
Fruchtblase	amnion	gelblich	yellowish
Fruchtblasenpunktion	amniocentesis	Gelbsucht	jaundice
Fruchtgetränk	fruit squash	Gelegenheit	opportunity
Fruchtwasser	amniotic fluid	gelegentlich	occasional(ly)
Frühdienst	early shift	Gelenk	joint
Frühgeborenes	premature	Gelenkkopf	condyle
frühreif	premature	gemäß	according to
Fügung	coincidence	gemein	vicious
fühlen	to feel	Gemeinde	community
führen	to conduct, to lead	Gemeindepflege	community care
Führung	leadership	gemeinsam	common(ly)
Fürsorgepfleger	district nurse	Gemisch	mixture
Furunkel	boil	genau	accurately
Fußwurzel(knochen)	tarsal	geneigt sein zu	to tend towards
füttern	to feed	Genesung	convalescence, healing, revocery
Gallenfarbstoff	bilirubin	gerade	straight
Gallenkolik	biliary colics	geringschätzig	contemptuous
Gallensteine	gallstones	Gerinnungsstörung	coagulation defect
Gänsehaut	goose flesh	Gerüchte	hearsay
ganzheitliche Krankenpflege	holistic nursing	gesamt	overall, entire
gastrointestinal	gastroinestinal	Gesamtorganismus betreffend	systemic
Gattung	species	Gesäß	buttocks
Gaze	gauze	geschehen	to occur
Gebärmutter	uterus	Geschöpf	creature
geben	to give	Geschwindigkeit	rate, speed
Geburtshelfer	obstetric nurse	Geschwür	ulcer
Geburtshilfliche Abteilung	obstetric department	Gesetz	Act, law, statute
		Gesetzgebung	legislation
geeignet	appropriate, suitable	Gesichtszug	feature
Gefahr	threat	gestatten	to allow

German	English	German	English
Gesundheitsamt	Department of Health (DoH)	gütig	charitable
Gesundheitsfürsorge	health care	Haarfollikel	hair follicle
Gesundheitszustand	health status	haben	to have
Gesundsein	wellness	Halluzination	vision
Getreideprodukte	cereals	Hals	neck, throat
getrennt durch	seperated by	Halsschlagader	carotid artery
gewinnen	to win, to gain, to derive	halten	to hold
		halten für	to deem
gewitzt	smart	Haltung	attitude, position
Gewohnheit	habit	Hämatologie	haematology
gewöhnlich	usually	Hämaglobin	haemoglobin
Gift	poison, venom	Hämophilie	haemophilia
giftig	poisonous, toxic	Hämorrhagie	haemorrhage
Gips	plaster (of Paris)	Hämorrhoiden	piles
glatt	smooth	Handbuch	manual
Glaube	belief	handeln	to deal
glauben	to believe	Handgriff	handgrip
gleich	equivalent	Handschuh	glove
Gleichartigkeit	similarity	Handtuch	bath blanket (USA), towel (UK)
gleichgültig	indifferent		
gleichmäßig	uniform	Handwagen	trolley
gleichwertig	equivalent	Handwurzel	wrist
gleiten	to slide, to slip	Handwurzelknochen	carpal
Gliedmaße	limb	hängen	to hang
Gonorrhoe	clap	harmlos	harmless
graben	to dig	Harnlassen	micturition
Gran	grain	hart	hard
Granulum	granule	Haube	cap
Graphik	graphic chart	Haupt-	main, principal
graphisch	graphic	hauptsächlich	primarily, principal
Grindflechte	impetigo	Hausbesuch	domiciliary
Grippe	flu	zum Haushalt gehörend	domestic
Großbuchstabe	capital letter		
großer Zeh	big toe	Haushaltshilfe	home help
großziehen	to raise	häuslich	domestic
Grund	cause	hauswirtschaftlicher Dienst	housekeeping department
der Grund sein für	to account for		
gründen	to establish, to launch	Hautentzündung	dermatitis
grundlegende Fragen	fundamental issues	Hautfalten	skin folds
gründlich	thourough(ly), rigorous	Hautfarbe	skin colour
		Hautkrankheit	skin disorder
Grundprinzip	rationale	Hautmal	spot
gurgeln	to gargle	Hebamme	midwife
Gurgelwasser	gargle	heben	to heave, to raise
Gurt	strap	Hefe	yeast
Guß	mould	Heftpflaster	adhesive plaster
gut gekleidet	well-dressed	Heil-	remedial
Güte	charity	Heilanzeige	indication
gutgläubig	trusting	heilend	remedial

German	English	German	English
Heilung	healing	Inkubator	incubator (UK), isolette (USA)
Heilverfahren	cure		
Heimlich-Griff	Heimlich manouvre	Innenknöchel	medial malleolus
heiser	thick	insbesondere	particularly
helfen	to accomodate	Inspektion	inspection
hell	clear	Insuffizienz	failure
hemmen	to arrest	integrieren	to integrate
Herausforderung	challenge	interagieren	to interact
herausgeben	to edit	Intervention	intervention
hervorheben	to emphasize, to high-light	Invalide	cripple
		inventarisieren	to list
Herzinsuffizienz	CHF		
Herzmassage	cardiac massage	Jahrzehnt	decade
Herzschlag	heartbeat	jämmerlich	mournful
Herzstillstand	cardiac arrest	Jochbein	zygomatic bone
Herzversagen	heart failure	Jod	iodine
Hilfe	relief		
Hilfs-	ancillary	Kahler-Krankheit	multiple myeloma
Hinterhauptsbein	occipital bone	Kaiserschnitt	Caesarean section
Hintern	bum	Kaliumpermanganat	potassium perman-ganate
hinwegsehen	to overlook		
Hinweis	indication	kämpfen	to fight
hinweisen	to indicate	Kardiologie	cardiology
hinzufügen	to add	Katastrophe	disaster
hinzuzählen	to add	kauen	to chew
HNO	ear-nose-throat (ENT)	kaufen	to buy
hochziehen	to raise	kaustisch	caustic
Hodgkin-Krankheit	Hodgkin's disease	Kehle	throat
Höhe	height	Kehlkopf	larynx
Höhle	cavity	Keim	germ
Höhlung	cavity	Kennzeichen	character, feature
Homöopathie	homeopathy	kennzeichnend	specific
hören	to hear	Keuchhusten	pertussis, whooping cough
Hornhaut	cornea		
hübsch	pretty	Kiefer	jaw
Hüfte	hip	Kieferknochen	jaw bone
Hypertrophie	hypertrophy	Kinderbettchen	crib
Hypnotherapie	hypnotherapy	Kinderstation	paediatric ward, pae-diatric department
ignorieren	to ignore	Kindertageshort	nursery
Immunisierung	immunization	Kinderwagen	perambulator, pram
Immunsystem	immune system	Kinderzimmer	nursery
Impfstoff	vaccine	kippen	to tilt
Impuls	impulse	Kissen	pillow
In-vitro-Befruchtung	in vitro fertilization	klagen	to complain
Inch	inch	Klaps	slap
Informationen	data	klar	apparent, clear
Inhalt	contents	Klarheit	clarity
Inkubationszeit	incubation period	Kleidungsstück	garment
		Kleinbuchstaben	lower case

German	English	German	English
kleiner Finger	little finger	Körpersprache	body language
kleiner werden	to shrink	Körpertemperatur	body temperature
kleiner Zeh	little toe, fifth toe	kostal	costal
Kleinteil	minute particle	kosten	to cost
Klingelknopf	bell push, signal cord	Kosten	expenditures
klingeln	ro ring	Kraft	strength
klinische Erfahrung	clinical experience	Kräfteschwund	marasmus
Klistier	enema	krank werden	to fall ill
klopfen	to tap	kränken	to offend
Klopfen	throbbing	Krankenbahre	stretcher
kneifen	to pinch	Krankengeschichte	case history
Knie	knee	Krankengymnast	physiotherapist
Kniekehle	popliteal space	Krankenpflege	nursing care
knien	to kneel	-kranker	sufferer
Kniescheibe	patella	Krankheit	ailment, illness, disease
Knöchel	ankle		
Knochenmark	bone marrow	Krankheitserreger	germ
Knopf	button	Krankheitsverlauf	course of a disease
knöpfen	to button	Kreuzbein	sacrum
Knorpel	cartilage	kriechen	to creep
kochen	to boil	Kropf	goitre, struma
Kohlehydratstoffwechsel	carbohydrate metabolism	Krüppel	cripple
		kühlen	to cool
kollabieren	to collapse	Kummer	heartache
Kollege	co-worker	kündigen	to quit
Komfort	comfort	künstliche Beatmung	artificial ventilation
kommen	to come	Kunststoff	synthetic
Kommentar	comment	Kurve	(graphic) chart
komplizierter Bruch	compound fracture	Kurzatmigkeit	shortness of breath
Kompresse	pad	kurze Hose	slacks (USA)
Kondition	condition	Kwashiokor	kwashiokor
Konsens	consensus		
konservieren	to preserve	Laborant	medical scientist
konsumieren	to consume	Labortest	laboratory test
Kontraktur	contracture	in der Lage sein	to be capable of
Kontrolle	CK	Lähmung	paralysis
kontrollieren	to control, to monitor	Laken	sheet
Kontrolliste	checklist	längerer Zeitraum	prolonged period
kontrovers	controversial	Langzeit-	long term
konvertieren	to convert	lassen	to leave, to let
konzentrieren	to focus	Laufstuhl	walker
Kopfschmerz	headache	lauschen	to eavesdrop
Korn	grain	laut	noisy
Körnchen	granule	läuten	to ring
Körper	body	Leberschädlichkeit	hepatotoxicity
Körperbild	body-image	Leck	leakage
Körperflüssigkeiten	body fluids	Leerdarm	jejunum
Körpergewebe	body tissue	legen	to lay, to put
körperliche Untersuchung	physical examination	lehnen	to lean
		lehren	to teach

German	English	German	English
leiden an	to suffer from	Material	equipment
Leidender	sufferer	Materie	matter
leihen	to lend	medial	medial
Leihmutterschaft	surrogacy	Medizinalassistent	houseman
Leinen	linen	medizinische Untersu-chung	check-up
Leistengegend	groin		
leiten	to conduct	medizinischer Assis-tent	practice nurse
leitend	ruling		
Leiter	administrator	Mehrheit	majority
Leiter des Pflegedienstes	nursing officer	meinen	to mean
		Meinungsumfrage	poll
Leitung	conduction, leadership	meistverwendet	most commonly
		Membrane	membrane
Lende	loin	Menge	amount, quantity
Lepra	leprosy	Menstruation	flow
lernen	to learn	Merkmal	feature
lesen	to read	messen	to measure
lieber mögen	to prefer	Messung	measurement
liefern	to deliver, to supply	Milchsekretion	lactation
liegen	to lie	Milz	spleen
Ligamentum	ligament	Minderbegabter	subnormal
Linctus	linctus	Mischung	mixture
lindern	to alleviate, to relieve	Missbrauch	abuse
Linderung	ease	misstrauisch	suspicious
Lob	praise	mithören	to listen in on
lobend	laudatory	Mittel	means, resource
logische Grundlage	rationale	Mittel-	medial
Logopädie	speech therapy	Mittelfinger	middle finger
Lohn	wages	Mittelfußknochen	metatarsals
lösen	to dislodge, to solve	Mittelhandknochen	metacarpals
Lösung	solution	Mittelohrentzündung	otitis media
Luftröhre	trachea, windpipe	Mitternacht	midnight
Luftwege	air passages, air way	Mitwirkung	contribution
Lungenembolie	PE	Müdigkeit	tiredness
Lustlosigkeit	apathy	mühsam	laboured
		Mull	gauze
machen	to make	Mumps	mumps
Magen	stomach	Mund-zu-Mund-Beatmung	kiss of life
Magen-Darm-	gastrointestinal		
Magenentzündung	gastritis	mündlicher Bericht	oral report
Magenpförtner	pylorus	Mundsoor	thrush
Mal	mark	Murmel	marble
Mangel	deficiency	Muskel	muscle
mangelhaft	vicious	Muskelatrophie	muscular waist
Manipulation	manipulation	Muskelfaser	muscle fibre
manuell	manual	Muster	sample, pattern
Marmor	marble	Mutterschaft	maternity, motherhood
Masern	measles		
Maß	degree, measurement		
Maßnahme	intervention, measure	Nabelschnur	umbilical cord

German	English	German	English
nachfolgend	subsequent	notwendigerweise	necessarily
Nachlassen	lessening	Notwendigkeit	need
nachlässig	disorderly	nüchtern	sober (Alkohol), NPO (Nahrung)
Nachtdienst	night shift		
Nachteil	disadvantage	Nutzen	benefit
Nachthemd	gown		
Nachtschränkchen	bedside table	Oberarmknochen	humerus
Nachttisch mit Klapp- vorrichtung	over-bed table	Oberfläche	surface
		Oberhemd	shirt
Nacken	nape of the neck	Oberkiefer	maxilla
Nagelbürste	nail brush	Oberkörper	upper body
nähen	to sew, to stitch	Oberschenkel	thigh
Nährstoffe	nutrients	Oberschenkelknochen	femur
Nahrung	nourishment	Oberseite	upper end
Naht	stitch	objektiv	objective
Narbe	mark	obwohl	although
Nasenloch	nostril	Ödem	oedema
Nasensonde	nasal cannula, naso- gastric tube (NG)	offensichtlich	apparent, obvious
		öffentliche Gesundheit	public health
nass machen	to wet	öffentlicher Platz	public place
Naturheilkunde	herbalism	Öffnung	outlet
Neben-	ancillary	oft	often
Nebenwirkung	side effect	Ohnmacht	faint
nehmen	to take	ohnmächtig werden	to faint
zu sich nehmen	to ingest	Ohrthermometer	aural thermometer
neigen	to tilt	Onkologie	oncology
Nekrose	gangrene	Oophorektomie	oophorectomy
Nerv	nerve	OP	operating theatre
Nervenentzündung	neuritis	OP-Schürze	gown
auf den neuesten Stand bringen	to update	OP-Schwester	theatre nurse
		Operation	surgery
Neugeborenes	newborn	sich einer Operation unterziehen	to undergo surgery
Neurochirurgie	neurosurgery		
Neurologie	neurology	Opfer	casualty, victim
neutralisieren	to counteract	ordnen	to arrange
nicht reanimieren	DNR	Orthopädie	orthopaedics
nichtteilnehmende Be- obachtung	non participant obser- vation	Osteopathie	osteopathy
		oxidieren	to oxidize
niedlich	cute	Oxygenation	oxygenation
Niere	kidney		
Niereninsuffizienz	renal failure	packen	to seize
Nierenschale	kidney tray	Pantoffeln	slippers
Niveau	level	parasitär	parasitic
NMR-Tomographie	magnet resonance imaging (MRI)	parasitisch	parasitic
		passen	to suit
Notaufnahme	emergency depart- ment	passend	suitable
		passieren	to happen
Notfall	emergency	Pastille	lozenge
Notfallabor	urgent laboratory	Pathologie	pathology
nötig	necessary	peinlich	embarrassing

German	English	German	English
Peitschenwurm	whipworm	prüfen	to audit
Pensionierung	retirement	Psychiatrische Einrichtung	mental clinic
peptisches Ulkus	peptic ulcer		
Perineum	perineum	Psychotherapie	psychotherapy
Perkussion	percussion	Puffotter	puff adder
Personal	staff	Puls	pulse
Pest	plague	Pulsschlag	pulse
pflanzlicher Organismus	vegetable life	Punkt	full stop, point
		Pustel	spot
Pflegeleiter	charge nurse		
Pflegemutter	nursing mother	Qual	distress, ordeal
Pflegeplan	nursing plan	quälen	to pinch
Pfleger 2. Grades	enrolled nurse (EN)	Qualifikation	qualification
Pfleger Erste Hilfe	A & E nurse	Quelle	source, resource
Pfleger für Kinderpflege	sick children's nurse (RSCN)	quer	transverse
		Quotient	ratio
Pfleger in der Intensivpflege	IC nurse		
		Rachen	throat
Pfleger, der Hausbesuche macht	health visitor	Rachitis	rickets
		Radial-	radial
Phenylketonurie	phenylketonuria	radioaktiv	radioactive
Physik	physics	Radius	radial, radius
Physiotherapie	physiotherapy	Röntgenabteilung	X-ray department
Pilz	fungus, mushroom	rasch	smart
Pinzette	tweezers	Rasseln	rale (crepitation)
Plan	scheme	sich keinen Rat wissen	to be at loss
Plastische Chirurgie	plastic surgery	raten	to guess
Plauderei	chat	reagieren	to respond
plötzlicher Anfall	seizure	Reaktionsvermögen	responsiveness
Pochen	throbbing	Reanimation	resuscitation
Poliklinik	out-patient	reduzieren	to reduce
Polster	pad	Reflexzonentherapie	reflexology
Position	position	Regel	rule
potentiell	potential	regelmäßig	frequently
Präposition	preposition	registrieren	to register
präventive Ausbildung	preventative teaching	regulieren	to adjust
Praxis	practice	reiben	to rub
präzise	accurately	reich	well-off, rich, wealthy
Präzision	conciseness	Reihenuntersuchung	survey
preiswert	cheap	reinigen	to clean, to cleanse
pressen	to press	Reinigung	defecation
primäre Lebenszeichen	vital signs	reißen	to tear
		Reißverschluss	zip
Probe	trial, specimen (Gewebe, Blut, Urin)	reiten	to ride
		reizen	to irritate
		Rekonvaleszenz	convalescence
prophylaktisch	prophylactic	Rektum	rectum
Prostata	prostate gland	rennen	to run
protestieren	to object	reparieren	to repair
Protozoen	protozoa	Replikation	replication

German	English	German	English
Ressourcen	resources	scharf	cutting
Retrospektive	restrospective	schätzen	to estimate
Rezept	prescription	schauen	to watch
richten auf	to adress	schaukeln	to rock
Richter	judge, Justice	Schaumstoffmatratze	eggcrate matress
richtig	appropriate, properly	scheiden	to separate
Richtlinie	rule, guideline	scheinen	to shine
in Richtung	towards	Scheitelbein	parietal
riechen	to smell	Schema	scheme, pattern
Riemen	strap	Schere	scissors
Ringfinger	ring finger	Schichtdienst arbeiten	to work in shifts
Rippen betreffend	costal	schick	smart
Rist	instep	schieben	to push, to slip
Röhrchen	straw	Schienbein	tibia
Röntgen	radiology	schießen	to shoot
Röntgenaufnahme	X-ray	Schilddrüse	thyroid gland
rotieren	to rotate	Schimmel	fungus, mould
Rückbildung	involution	schlafen	to sleep
rückblickend	retrospective	Schlaflosigkeit	insomnia
Rücken	back	Schlag	slap
Rückenabreibung	back rub	Schlagader	artery
Rückenmark	spinal cord	Schlaganfall	stroke
Rückfall	relapse	schlagen	to beat, to strike
Rückgang	decrease	Schlangenbiss	snake bite
rückwärts	backwards	schlau	cute
Ruhestand	retirement	Schlauchbinde	stockinette
ruhig	quiet	schlechte Ohren	poor hearing
ruhiger werden	to settle down	Schleim	phlegm
Rumpf	trunk	Schleimabsonderung	mucus secretion
rutschen	to slip	Schleimhäute	mucous membranes
		schließen	to shut
sachlich	factual, objective	schlucken	to swallow
sagen	to say, to tell	Schlüsselbegriff	key word
sägen	to saw	Schlüsselbein	clavicle
Salbe	ointment	schlüssig	conclusive
sammeln	to gather, to collect	schmal	narrow
Satzung	statute	Schmerz	distress, pain
Sauerstoff	oxygen	Schmerz zufügen	to hurt
Sauerstoffanreiche- rung	oxygenation	schmutzig	soiled
		Schnabeltasse	feeding cup
Sauerstoffmangel	hypoxia	schnalzen	to snap
Saugen	suction	Schnarchen	snoring
Saugwirkung	suction	schneiden	to cut
Schädel	cranium, skull	schnell	rapid(ly)
Schaden	harm	schnippen	to snap
schädlich	injurious	Schnitt	cut, cutting, incision
Schafsfell	sheepskin	Schnittwunde	incision
Schambein	pubis	schräg stellen	to tilt
Schambeinknorpel- fuge	symphysis pubis	schreiben	to write
		schreien	to scream

| --- | --- | --- | --- |
Schuhlöffel	shoehorn	sicher	firm(ly)
schulen	to train	sichere Umgebung	safe environment
Schulkrankenpfleger	school nurse	Sicherheitsnadel	safety pin
Schulter	shoulder	sicherstellen	to ensure
Schulterblatt	scapula, shoulder blade	sichtbar	visible
		Siedepunkt	boiling point
Schüttelfrost	chill	singen	to sing
schütteln	to shake	sinken	to sink
Schutz	guard	Sinusknoten	sinoatrial node
schwach	faint	Sitzbein	ischium
Schwäche	weakness	sitzen	to sit
schwache Augen	poor eyesight	Skorbut	scurvy
Schwächung	impairment	Slip	briefs (UK), panties
schwanger	pregnant	so schnell wie möglich	a.s.a.p.
schwanger werden	to conceive	sofort	immediately
Schwanz	tail	Sog	suction
schwellen	to swell	Sonde	probe
Schwellung	swelling	Sorge	distress
schwerfällig	laboured	sorgen für	to supply
Schwertfortsatz	xiphoid process	sich Sorgen machen	to worry
Schwester	sister	Sozialarbeit	social services
schwierig	hard	soziale Sicherheit	social security
Schwierigkeiten mit	difficulties in	spannen	to stretch, to tighten
Schwimmbecken	pool	Spannung	tension
schwimmen	to swim	Spätdienst	back shift
Schwindel	dizziness	Speiche	radius
Schwinden	disappearance	Speiseröhre	oesophagus
Schwindsucht	consumption	spezifisch	specific
schwingen	to swing	an der Spitze stehen	to head
schwitzen	to sweat	Splitter	sliver, splinter
sehen	to see	Sprachbarriere	language barrier
Sehkraft	vision	sprechen	to speak
Sehne	tendon	Sprechstunde	surgery hours
Sehvermögen	sight	Sprechstunde abhalten	to run surgery
Seil	rope		
sein	to be	Sprechvermögen	speech
Seitenlage	lateral position	springen	to spring
seitlich	lateral	Spritze	syringe
Sekretion	secretion	Sprosspilz	yeast
Selbstachtung	self-esteem	spucken	to spit
Selbsthilfe	self-help skills	stabil	firm(ly)
Selbstmord	suicide	stabile Seitenlage	recovery position
Selbstmordversuch	parasuicide	Stabilität	stability
selten	rare	Stachel	spine
sensibel	sensitive	standhalten	to withstand
separat	separately	Standpunkt	attitude
setzen	to put, to set	Stange	bar
Seuche	plague	Stärke	severity, strength
sexuelle Belästigung	sexual advances	Station	ward
Sichelzellenanämie	sickle cell anaemia	Stationsschwester	sister

German	English	German	English
Staub	dust	stürmen	to storm
stechen	to sting	Substanz	substance
stechender Schmerz	stabbing pain	suchen	to seek
stehen	to stand	Sucht	habit
stehlen	to steal	Symmetrie	symmetry
Steifheit	stiffness	Symptom	symptom
steigen	to rise	synthetisch	synthetic
steigern	to enhance	systolischer Druck	systolic pressure
Stein	calculus		
Steinstaublunge	silicosis	Tablette	lozenge
Steißbein	coccyx	Taille	waist
Steißlage	breech presentation	Taschentuch	hanky
stellen	to put, to set	tatsächlich	factual
Stelleninhaber	post-holder	Tau	rope
sterben	to pass away	Taubheit	deafness
Sterbesakramente	last rites	Tee	tea
Stich	stitch	Teewagen	trolley
Stickstoff	nitrogen	in Teile zerlegt	fragmented
stickstoffhaltig	nitrogenuous	teilen	to divide, to share
still	quiet	teilweise	partial
stillen	to breast-feed	Telegramm	cable
stillende Mutter	nursing mother	Test	trial
stinken	to stink	These	thesis
Stock	bar	Thyroxin	thyroxine
Stoff	matter, substance	Tibia	tibia
Stoffwechsel	metabolism	tief schlafen	to be sound asleep
Stoffwechselstörung	metabolic disorder	tiefgehend	thourough(ly)
stören	to bother	Tier	creature
störend	disturbing	toben	to storm
Störung	defect, disorder, disturbance, failure	Toilettenartikel	toiletries
		Tollwut	rabies
Stoß	thrust	Tonsillenentfernung	tonsillectomy
stoßen	to strike, to push	Tortur	ordeal
Strafe	punishment	töten	to slay
straffen	to tighten	TPR-Werte	TPR values
Strahlung	radiation	tragen	to bear, to wear (Kleidung)
Strang	rope		
strecken	to stretch	Träger	vector
streiten	to fight	Traktion	traction
Strenge	severity	Transfer	transfer
Strick	rope	Transpiration	perspiration
stricken	to knit	transversal	transverse
Strickjacke	cardigan	Trapez	trapeze
strikt	rigorous	Trauer	grief
Strom	electricity, electric current, current, flow	Trauerfall	bereavement
		Trauma	trauma
Strömung	current	träumen	to dream
Strumpfhose	pantyhose (USA), tights	traurig	mournful
		treffen	to hit, to strike, to meet
Stuhlgang	stools		

treibend	afloat	Ulkus	ulcer
trennen	to separate	umdrehen	to turn
Trikotstrumpf	stockinette	Umfang	spread
trinken	to drink	umfassend	comprehensive
Tropfinfusion	droplet method	umgeben	to surround
Trost	comfort	Umkehrung	reversal
trösten	to comfort	Umschlag	reversal
trotzdem	nevertheless	Umstände	circumstances
trüben	to thicken	umstritten	controversial
Tuch	cloth	umwandeln	to convert, to metabolize
Tücher	tissues		
tun	to do	umziehen	to change
zu tun haben mit	to be concerned with	Unabhängigkeit	independance
Typhus	typhoid fever	unangebracht	inappropriate
		unangemessen	inadequate
Übelkeit	nausea	Unannehmlichkeit	discomfort
Übelkeit verspüren	to feel queasy	unbedingt	necessarily
Überalterung	ageing population	unbegründet	ill-founded
Überblick	survey	uneigennützig	altruistic
überblicken	to overlook	unerträglich	intolerable
überdehnen	to overstrech	Unfähigkeit	inability
Überdosis	overdose	Unfruchtbarkeit	infertility
Übereinstimmung	agreement, consensus	ungefährlich	harmless
überfüllt	overcrowded	ungerecht	unfair
übergeben	to hand over	ungewöhnlich	unusual(ly)
sich übergeben	to be sick	Unglück	disaster
überleben	to survive	ungünstig	unfavourable
Übermaß	excess	unlauter	unfair
übermäßig	excessive	unmittelbar	promptly
Übermüdung	tiredness	unnötig	unnecessary
überprüfen	to review	Unordnung	disorder
überraschend	surprising(ly)	unpassend	improper, inappropriate
überreicht	presented		
überschreiten	to exceed	Unregelmäßigkeiten	irregularities
Überschuss	excess	Unsicherheit	uncertainty
übersehen	to ignore, to overlook	Unterarm	forearm
Übersicht	scheme, survey	unterbrechen	to interrupt
übersteigen	to exceed	unterbringen	to accomodate
übertragen	to transmit, to delegate	unterdrücken	to suppress
		unterdurchschnittlich	subnormal
Übertragung	transfer	untere Extremität	lower extremity
überwachen	to control, to monitor, to watch	Unterernährung	malnutrition
		Unterhemd	undershirt (USA), vest (UK)
überwältigen	to overcome		
überwinden	to overcome	Unterhose	underpants (UK)
überzeugen	to convince	Unterkiefer	mandible
überzeugend	conclusive	Unterkühlung	hypothermia
überziehen	to line	unterlassen	to omit
üblicherweise	usually	unterrichten	to teach
Übung	exercise	unterscheiden	to distinguish

German	English	German	English
Unterschenkelamputation	BKA	verbrauchen	to consume
		verbreiten	to spread
Unterschied	distinction, variance	Verbreitung	spread
unterstützen	to support, to back up	verbrennen	tu burn
Unterstützung	support	verbringen	to spend
untersuchen	to investigate, to poll, to examine, to explore	Verdauungstrakt	digestive tube, digestive tract
		verdeutlichen	to cast light on
Untersuchung	inspection, examination	verdicken	to thicken
		Verdoppelung	replication
Unterwäsche	underwear	verdrängen	to dislodge
unumkehrbar	irreversible	vereinbaren	to arrange
unveränderter Zustand	status quo	Vereinbarung	agreement, arrangement
unverantwortlich	irresponsible	vereinheitlichen	to standardise
Unvermögen	inability	sich vereinigen	to join
unverzüglich	immediately	Vereinigung	association
Unvollkommenheit	deficiency	vererben	to transmit
unwahr	false	Verfall	marasmus
Unwissenheit	ignorance	verfärben	to discolour
unzufrieden	dissatisfied	verfügbar	available
unzulänglich	inadequate	zur Verfügung stellen	to provide
Urinieren	micturition, urination	verführerisch	tempting
urinieren	to pass urine	vergessen	to forget
Urinuntersuchung	urine test	vergewaltigen	to violate
Urologie	urology	vergießen (Blut, Tränen)	to shed
Ursache	cause		
Urteil	judgement	Vergleich	simile
		Vergrößerung	enlargement
Vaginaluntersuchung	vaginal examination	verhalten	to behave
Vakuumextraktion	vacuum extraction	Verhalten	behaviour
Vektor	vector	menschliche Verhaltensmuster	human response pattern
Ventil	outlet	Verhältnis	ratio
verabreichen	to administer	verhandeln	to bargain
Verabreichung	administration	verhüten	to avoid, to prevent
verächtlich	contemptuous	verkaufen	to sell
Veränderung	alteration	verklemmen	to wedge
verantwortlich	responsible, accountable	Verlagerung	dislocation
verantwortlich sein	to be in charge	verlangen	to call for, to demand
Verantwortung	responsibility	Verlangen	desire
Verband	bandage, cloth	verlangen	to stipulate
verbergen	to hide	verlassen	to leave, to quit
verbessern	to improve	sich verlassen auf	to rely on
Verbesserung	improvement	Verlegenheit	embarrassement
verbieten	to forbid, to outlaw	Verlegung	transfer
verbinden	to connect, to join	verletzen	to hurt
verbinden mit	to link with	verletzt	injured
Verbindung	conjunction	Verletzung	harm, injury
Verbrauch	consumption	verlieren	to lose

German	English	German	English
verlockend	tempting	verwischen	to blur
Verlust	loss	verzehren	to consume
vermeiden	to avoid, to prevent	völlig	entirely
vermieten	to let	vollständige parente-	TPN
vermuten	to guess, to imagine	rale Ernährung	
Vermutung	presumption	vor	ahead
verordnen	to prescribe	voran	ahead
verrenken	to luxate	vorausgehend	previous
Verrenkung	dislocation	vorbereiten	to prepare
verringern	to reduce	vorbereitet	prepared
Versagen	failure	Vorbereitung	preparation
versammeln	to gather	vorenthalten	to withhold, to deprive
Versammlung	meeting		of
verschicken	to send	vorgeben	to pretend
Verschiedenheit	diversity	vorgelegt	presented
Verschlechterung	exacerbation	Vorhaben	intention
verschleiern	to blur	vorherrschend	ruling, predominant
Verschlimmerung	exacerbation	vorhersehbar	predictable
Verschluss	obstruction	vorkommen	to occur
verschmutzt	soiled	Vormilch	colostrum
Verschmutzung	pollution	vornehmen	to perform
verschreiben	to prescribe	vornüberbeugen	to bend over
verschütten	to spill	vorschlagen	to suggest
Verschwinden	disappearance	vorschreiben	to stipulate
versehentlich	accidental, inadver-	Vorsicht	caution
	tently	vorsichtig	careful(ly)
versenden	to send	Vorsteherdrüse	prostate gland
versichern	to assure, to insure	vorstellen	to imagine
Versicherung	assurance, insurance	Vorteil	advantage, benefit
versorgen	to look after	vorübergehend	temporary
Verstand	wit	vorübergehende Bes-	remission
verstauchen	to sprain	serung	
verstehen	to understand, to	vorwärts	forward
	grasp	vorzeitig	premature
verstoffwechseln	to metabolize	vorziehen	to prefer
Verstopfung	obstruction	Vorzug	preference
verstoßen gegen	to offend, to violate		
Versuch	trial	Waage	scales
versuchen	to attempt	wachsen	to grow
vertrauensvoll	trusting	Wade	calf
Vertraulichkeit	confidentiality	Wadenbein	fibula
verursachen	to generate	während	during
vervielfältigen	to multiply	Wahrheit	truth
Verwalter	administrator	wahrscheinlich	probably
Verwaltung	administration	Wand	wall
verwaschene Sprache	slurred speech	warten (Maschine)	to maintain
Verwendung	use	Wartezimmer	waitingroom
verwickeln	to involve	Wartungsabteilung	maintenance depart-
verwirrt	confused		ment
Verwirrung	disturbance	Wasserblase	blister

German	English	German	English
Wassergeburt	water-birth	Wochenfluss	lochia
Wasserstoffperoxid	hydrogen peroxide	Wohlbefinden	wellness
wechseln	to change, to vary	wohltätig	charitable
wechselwirken	to interact	wörtlich	literally
wecken	to wake	wund	sore
wegen	due to	wundgelegene Stelle	bedsore
Wegwerf-	disposable	Wundheilung	intention
Wehen	contractions, labour	Wunsch	desire
in den Wehen liegen	to labour	wünschen	to bid
weinen	to weep	würgen	to choke, to suffocate
Weiß der Augen	whites of the eyes	Wurzel	root
weitergeben	to hand over		
weiterleiten	to transmit	Xerophthalmie	xerophthalmia
weitverbreitet	common(ly)		
Weizenkeim	wheat germ	Z-Pfleger	mentally handicapped nurse (RNMH)
wenden	to turn		
werden	to become	Zahn	tooth
werfen	to cast, to throw	Zahn- und Kieferchirurgie	dental surgery
Werkzeug	tool		
Werturteil	value judgement	Zahnfleisch	gum
wertvoll sein	to be of value	Zahngesundheit	dental health
Weste	vest (USA)	Zangengeburt	forceps delivery
wetten	to bet	Zäpfchen	suppository
wichtig	significant, important	Zehe	toe
wichtig sein	to be of value	Zehenglied	phalanges
widersprechen	to conflict	Zeichen	sign
widerstehen	to withstand	zeichnen	to draw
widrig	unfavourable	Zeigefinger	forefinger, index finger
wie gewünscht	PRN	zeigen	to show
wieder aufnehmen	to readmit	Zeitspanne	time span
wieder einweisen	to readmit	Zeitumfang	time span
Wiederausrichtung	realignment	Zellteilung	division of cells
Wiederbelebung	resuscitation	zentrales Nervensystem	central nervous system
wieder erkennen	to recognize		
wiederherstellen	to restore	Zentralküche	diatery department
wiederholen	to repeat, to reiterate	zerknittert	wrinkled
wiederholt	repeatedly	zerreißen	to rupture
wiegen	to rock	zerren	to sprain
willkürlich	randomly	zerstören	to destroy
winden	to wind	zeugen	to beget, to generate
Wirbel	vertebra	Zeugnis	qualification
Wirbelsäule	vertebral column	ziehen	to draw
wirksam	effective(ly)	Ziehen	traction
Wirksamkeit	efficacy	Ziel	goal, objective, aim
Wirkungsbereich	radius	ziemlich	fairly
wischen	to wipe	Zischen	zip
wissen	to know	zitieren	to quote
wissenschaftlich	scientific	zittern	to shiver
Witz	wit	züchten	to reproduce
witzig	witty	Zufall	coincidence

German	English	German	English
zufällig	accidental(ly), randomly	zusammenziehen	to contract
		zusätzlich	supplementary
zufrieden mit	content with	zusätzliche Beratung	second opinion
Zug	traction	zuschließen	to lock
Zugang	access	Zustand	status
zugestehen	to permit	Zustellung	delivery
zugrunde liegen	to underlie	zustimmen	to consent
Zulassungsanforderungen	entry level	Zweck	purpose
		zweideutig	ambiguous
Zunahme	increase	Zweifel	doubt
zunehmend	progressive	zweifelhaft	doubtful, dubious
Zungenentzündung	glossitis	Zwerchfell	diaphragm
zurückblicken	to review	Zwillinge	twins
zurückhalten	to retain	zwingen	to compel, to force
zurückkommen	to return	zwischenmenschlich	interpersonal
zurückweisen	to refuse, to reject	Zwölffingerdarm	duodenum
Zusammenarbeit	collaboration	zyklisch	cyclical
Zusammentreffen	conjunction		

Key

1.1

1-b, **2**-d, **3**-a, **4**-d, **5**-a, **6**-b, **7**-b, **8**-d, **9**-c

1.2

1 medical scientist
2 training
3 psychiatric hospital/mental clinic
4 to broaden
5 qualifications

6 to separate
7 mental problems
8 congenital
9 nursing assistant/ancillary nurse
10 grade

1.4

1-i, **2**-f, **3**-a, **4**-d, **5**-j, **6**-g, **7**-b, **8**-k, **9**-e, **10**-h, **11**-c

1.5

1 expenditure (l. 30)
2 insurance (l. 9/10)
3 dissatisfied (l. 35)
4 equity (l. 33)
5 benefit (l. 13)

6 extended (l. 18)
7 charitable (l. 21)
8 adoption (l. 28)
9 social security (l. 3)
10 covers (l. 10)

1.7

1 Write to this hospital if you are looking for a new job.
2 I am applying for the post of charge nurse.
3 This student nurse is getting on my nerves.

4 The physiotherapist is doing exercises with him.
5 The speech therapist is trying to improve her communication skills.

1.8

1 to
2 from
3 at
4 by
5 in

6 in
7 in
8 from
9 by
10 with

11 by
12 with
13 in
14 at
15 in

16 of
17 in
18 to
19 by
20 with/in

Unit 1

1.9

1-b, **2**-e, **3**-g, **4**-a, **5**-h, **6**-f, **7**-d, **8**-i, **9**-j, **10**-c

1.10

1	is always complaining/always complains	**8**	smokes secretly/is secretly smoking
2	freezes	**9**	usually comes
3	is bleeding	**10**	makes
4	is leaving	**11**	is checking
5	arrives	**12**	is behaving
6	is making	**13**	always takes
7	do you think	**14**	live
		15	burn/burning

1.11

1	paediatrician	**8**	oncologist
2	haematologist	**9**	orthopaedist
3	radiologist	**10**	gynaecologist
4	rheumatologist	**11**	psychiatrist
5	ophthalmologist	**12**	surgeon
6	obstetrician	**13**	geriatrician
7	cardiologist	**14**	dermatologist

Unit 2

2.1

1 false, **2** false, **3** true, **4** true, **5** true, **6** false, **7** false.

2.3

The man was probably admitted to a urology ward.

2.4

a palpation
b auscultation
c inspection
d percussion

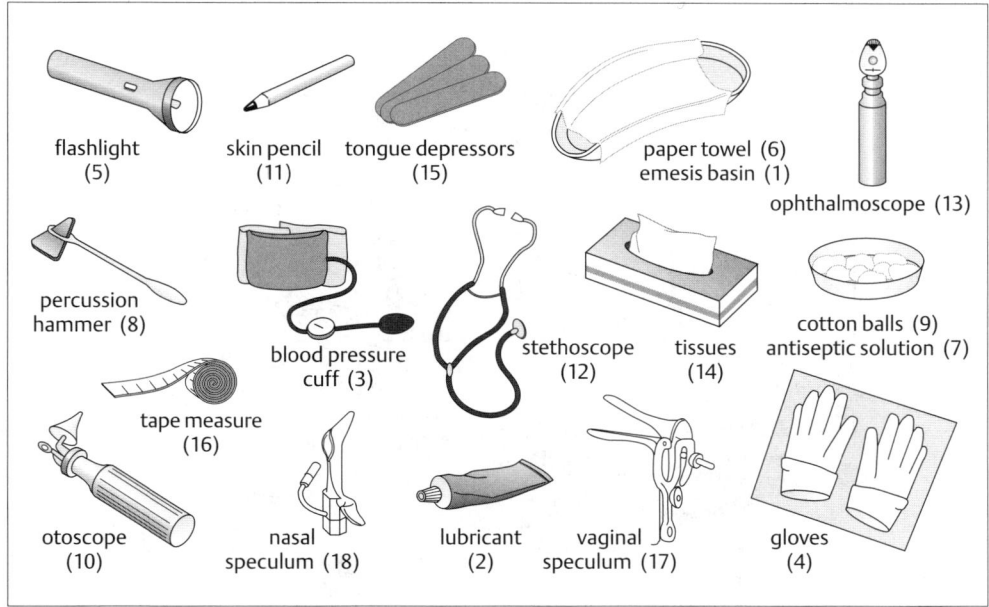

flashlight
(5)

skin pencil
(11)

tongue depressors
(15)

paper towel (6)
emesis basin (1)

ophthalmoscope (13)

percussion
hammer (8)

blood pressure
cuff (3)

stethoscope
(12)

tissues
(14)

cotton balls (9)
antiseptic solution (7)

tape measure
(16)

otoscope
(10)

nasal
speculum (18)

lubricant
(2)

vaginal
speculum (17)

gloves
(4)

2.5

1	fell	**6**	was
2	saw	**7**	died
3	injected	**8**	rose
4	am, am/was, was	**9**	asks/asked
5	visits/visited	**10**	fell

2.6

1 He slept soundly last night.

2 The patients went home for the weekend.

3 I heard a strange noise in his room.

4 The old lady ate all of her porridge.

5 He drank two glasses of milk at breakfast.

Unit 2

2.7

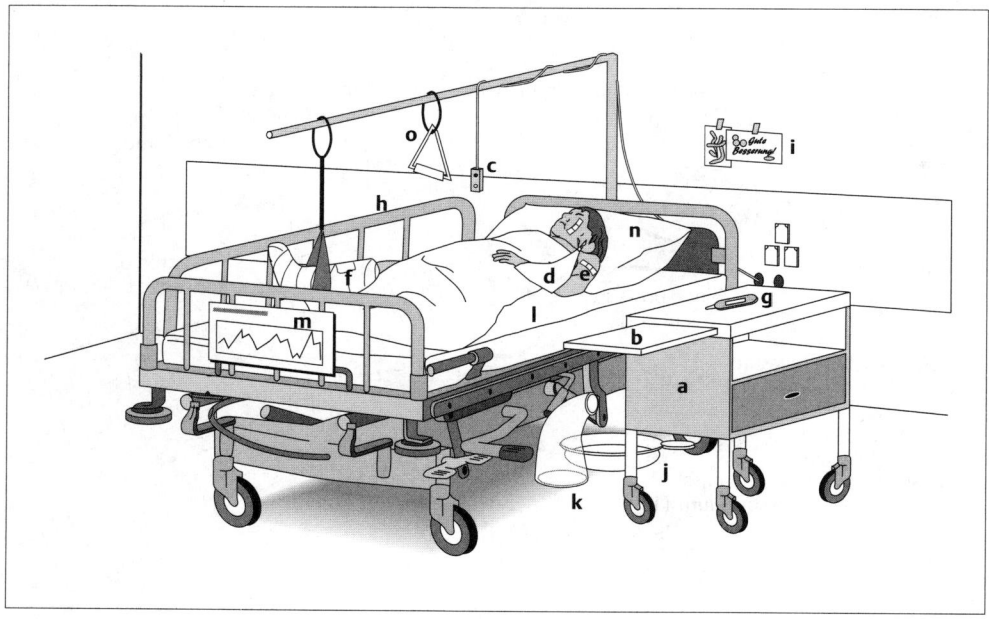

2.8

1 paediatric epartment/ward/unit
2 obstetric department/ward
3 renal unit
4 emergency department (USA)/A & E (UK) (casualty)
5 theatre

6 X-ray department
7 oncology dept./ward
8 pulmonary dept./ward/unit
9 ENT dept./ward
10 surgical dept./ward

2.9

1-p, **2**-e, **3**-a, **4**-k, **5**-c, **6**-m, **7**-g, **8**-b, **9**-q, **10**-d, **11**-n, **12**-f, **13**-j, **14**-h, **15**-i, **16**-o, **17**-l

2.10

1 regained
2 take
3 lost
4 does/makes
5 is measuring

6 hold
7 is suffering
8 get
9 feel
10 caught

2.11

1	true	**6**	false
2	false	**7**	true
3	true	**8**	false
4	true	**9**	true
5	false	**10**	true

3.1

1-b, **2**-c, **3**-a, **4**-d, **5**-b, **6**-a, **7**-d, **8**-b, **9**-c, **10**-a, **11**-d, **12**-a, **13**-b, **14**-c, **15**-c

3.2

1	assigned to	**6**	agitated
2	back shift	**7**	to wet a bed
3	fortunately	**8**	to rush
4	early shift	**9**	a bedpan
5	to wander	**10**	to increase

3.3

M 1, 4, 7, 11, 13
B 3, 10, 15, 17, 20
D 8, 14, 18
A 2, 5, 6, 9, 12, 16, 19

3.4

1-b, **2**-h, **3**-g, **4**-f, **5**-a, **6**-d, **7**-e, **8**-c

3.6

1	2-7-10
2	1-5-18
3	4-13-17
4	6-8-12
5	9-11-14
6	3-15-16

Unit 3

3.7

1	sleeve	**6**	to draw up
2	cardigan	**7**	shoehorn
3	bra	**8**	pantyhose (USA), tights (UK)
4	undershirt (USA), vest (UK)	**9**	to zip
5	slippers	**10**	garment

3.8

1	have lived	**6**	was born
2	were you	**7**	has (just) come in
3	lent	**8**	called
4	has been	**9**	did you see
5	checked	**10**	have been/were transferred

3.9

1 This hospital was built in the last century.
2 We have known her since she was a little girl.
3 I have checked him every hour/hourly.
4 I dropped a flask of blood yesterday.
5 Have you heard the bad news yet?

3.10

1-e, **2**-h, **3**-c, **4**-j, **5**-d, **6**-a, **7**-f, **8**-b, **9**-i, **10**-l, **11**-g, **12**-k

3.11

1 Is a heel protector used to ... No, it isn't used to ...
2 Should synthetic sheepskin be placed ... Yes, it should be placed ...
3 Does an egg-crate mattress ... Yes, it does add comfort ...
4 Does a bedcradle prevent ... No, it doesn't prevent ...
5 Is Sims' position ... Yes, it is ...
6 Does liquid food contain ... No, it doesn't contain ...
7 Should nauseous patients ... No, they shouldn't be nursed ...
8 Are patients usually ... Yes, they are usually placed ...
9 Are patients with ...Yes, they are often fed ...
10 Does a walker provide ... Yes, it does provide ...

1	insomnia	**5**	bedcradle	**9**	dry-clean	**13**	stertor
2	incontinence	**6**	cutlery	**10**	nightie	**14**	feeding cup
3	charge nurse	**7**	admission	**11**	procedure	**15**	ancillary nurse
4	kilogram	**8**	bedsores	**12**	observation		

4.1

1-f, **2**-j, **3**-a, **4**-b, **5**-c, **6**-d, **7**-e, **8**-g, **9**-h, **10**-i

4.2

1	hay fever	**4**	haemorrhoids
2	handkerchief	**5**	Antabuse
3	menopause		

4.3

1	relapse	**4**	complication
2	remission	**5**	convalescence
3	exacerbation		

4.4

1	the incubation period	**6**	headache	**13**	hereditary disease	**17**	industrial disease
2	germs	**7**	rash	**14**	deficiency disease	**18**	dust
3	fight	**8**	cancer	**15**	infections	**19**	chemical pollution
4	the immune system	**9**	AIDS	**16**	flu, mumps, measles	**20**	pneumoconiosis
5	diarrhoea	**10**	infection				
		11	transmitted				
		12	haemophilia				

4.5

1	shall/will help	**4**	shall/will try	**7**	shall go	**9**	should ask
2	will arrive	**5**	will be	**8**	will return	**10**	would help
3	will leave	**6**	will come				

Unit 4

4.6

1 The patient says that she will do it.
2 We shall/will give you a ring/call you.
3 The surgeon will operate on him to-morrow.
4 The vaccination will produce immunity to the disease.
5 He will soon be covered with a rash.

4.9

1-a, 2-e, 3-g, 4-b, 5-h, 6-d, 7-i, 8-j, 9-f, 10-c

4.10

1-e, 2-f, 3-i, 4-d, 5-h, 6-c, 7-a, 8-j, 9-g, 10-b

Unit 5

5.1

1 a tendency to behave in a particular way
2 in spite of that
3 lack of knowledge
4 to reduce the effect by opposite action
5 something clever and amusing
6 hollow tube into which liquid can be sucked
7 causing feelings of courage, hope and confidence
8 sad

5.2

1	immune	3	immunity	5	inherited	7	immunization
2	susceptible	4	born	6	developed	8	acquired

5.4

1	can/may	4	could/may/	6	shall/will		should
2	may/might		might	7	should	9	shall/will
3	must/need to	5	must/need to	8	ought to/	10	may

5.5

1 I will come and see you soon.
2 You should pay more attention.
3 You may go as soon as you are finished.
4 You ought to/should be more careful.
5 Could/can you press that button for me, please?

1	true	**4**	true	**7**	false	**9**	false
2	false	**5**	false	**8**	true	**10**	true
3	true	**6**	true				

5.7

1	iron deficiency (l. 33)	**10**	commissioned (l. 7)
2	jointly (l. 7)	**11**	anaemic (l. 11)
3	nutrients (l. 10)	**12**	balanced (l. 3)
4	educate (title)/(l. 50 inform)	**13**	consumed (l. 38)
5	DoH (l. 7)	**14**	reassuring (l. 29)
6	at the end of the day (l. 51)	**15**	confectionary (l. 23/24)
7	to take note (l. 18)	**16**	tooth decay (l. 46/47)
8	reiterated (l. 20)	**17**	concern (l. 36/37)
9	Ministry of Agriculture, Fisheries and Foods (l. 8/9)	**18**	fizzy drinks (l. 24)
		19	survey (l. 4)
		20	deprive (l. 55)

5.8

1	–	ground floor	–
2	–	–	mean
3	–	–	closet
4	Kinderwagen	–	–
5	–	–	barf
6	–	–	mad
7	–	–	elevator
8	–	–	diaper
9	null	–	–
10	–	traineeship	–
11	Universität	–	–
12	–	holiday	vacation
13	Abfalleimer	–	–
14	–	–	flashlight
15	Krankengeld	–	–
16	–	neighbours	neighbors
17	–	centre	–
18	–	cheque	check
19	Ehre	–	–
20	–	spilt	–

21	gerochen	–	–
22	–	–	gynecologist
23	–	haematology	–
24	–	orthopaedist	orthopedist
25	Programm	–	–
26	–	flavour	–
27	–	–	behavior

5.9

1	riboflavin		**9**	toxin
2	intramuscular		**10**	booster
3	breast milk		**11**	immunization
4	magnesium		**12**	health
5	incidence		**13**	antigen
6	dehydration		**14**	amino acids
7	hygiene		**15**	immunoglobulin
8	sugar lump			

6.1

1-c, **2**-d, **3**-a, **4**-d, **5**-a, **6**-c, **7**-d, **8**-a, **9**-c, **10**-a

6.2

1-g, **2**-k, **3**-l, **4**-i, **5**-b, **6**-n, **7**-r, **8**-c, **9**-s, **10**-p

6.3

1	true		**6**	true
2	false		**7**	false
3	false		**8**	false
4	true		**9**	true
5	false		**10**	true

6.4

1-b, **2**-f, **3**-s, **4**-g, **5**-o, **6**-t, **7**-k, **8**-c, **9**-m, **10**-a, **11**-i (j), **12**-j, **13**-l, **14**-r, **15**-n, **16**-h, **17**-p, **18**-q, **19**-d, **20**-e

1 pyjamas
2 spectacles/specs
3 teeth
4 potatoes
5 hospital buses

6 women
7 medicine(s)/medication/drugs
8 beliefs
9 shelves
10 baths

6.6

1 I cannot find the scissors.
2 The patients made little progress.
3 She dropped two knives.

4 This analysis uses three criteria.
5 Can you take these ladies to their room(s)?

6.7

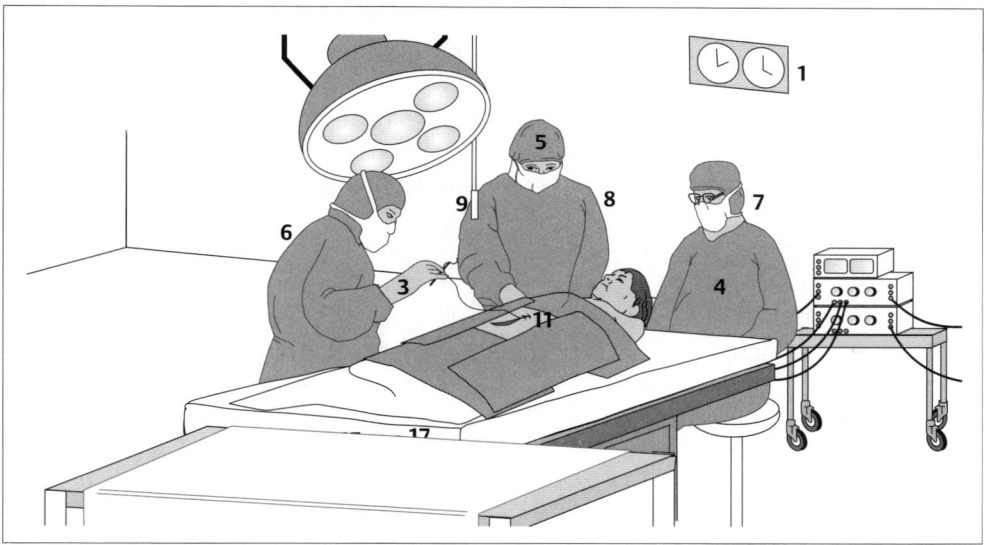

6.8

1 yes
2 at 6 o'clock in the morning
3 12 (= noon) in the morning
4 no
5 yes, a urine specimen

6 no
7 no
8 no
9 no
10 yes

Unit 6

6.9

1-i, **2**-c, **3**-f, **4**-a, **5**-b, **6**-g, **7**-h, **8**-j, **9**-d, **10**-e

6.10

1	medicines	**6**	allergic reactions
2	swallowed	**7**	prescribing
3	antacids	**8**	Jehovah's Witnesses
4	gastritis	**9**	blood
5	anticoagulants	**10**	consent

Unit 7

7.1

1-l, **2**-h, **3**-a, **4**-q, **5**-m, **6**-b, **7**-p, **8**-j, **9**-c, **10**-e, **11**-o, **12**-d, **13**-t, **14**-i, **15**-f, **16**-s, **17**-g, **18**-k, **19**-n, **20**-r

7.2

1 She had twins.
2 They hadn't noticed Kay was in a breech presentation.
3 By a drip.
4 By a Caesarean section. (USA: Cesarean birth)
5 No, breast-fed.

7.3

1 Caesarean section
2 contractions
3 conception
4 dilatation
5 forceps delivery
6 umbilical cord
7 amnion

7.5

1 This is the girl for whom the medicine was prepared.
2 Whose nappy is that?
3 I went to the midwife who/that was on call.
4 The milk which/that was diluted smelled mouldy/musty/stale.
5 Do you know who left this pram/baby carriage/buggy here?

1 true
2 true
3 false

4 false(?)
5 true

7.7

1-b, **2**-d, **3**-a, **4**-d, **5**-a, **6**-b, **7**-d, **8**-c, **9**-c

7.8

1 to call off
2 to call for
3 to call in/by/round/on
4 to look after
5 to look out
6 to look up
7 to send for
8 to send off
9 to turn up
10 to turn out

11 to turn down/away
12 to turn off
13 to go off
14 to go on
15 to go up
16 to go down
17 to bring over
18 to bring round
19 to bring back
20 to bring on/about

7.9

1 burp
2 ultrasound
3 perineum
4 contraction

5 isolette
6 episiotomy
7 afterbirth
8 maternity

9 infection
10 cradle
11 dilatation

12 neonate
13 pregnancy
14 breastfeeding

8.1

Unit 8

1-c, **2**-d, **3**-a, **4**-a, **5**-d, **6**-b, **7**-b, **8**-d, **9**-c

8.2

1 Wartezimmer
2 ersticken
3 Murmel

4 Bauch
5 Versuche
6 Wagen

7 Krankenbahre
8 nähen
9 nüchtern

10 in Ohnmacht
fallen

Unit 8

8.3

1	true	**4**	true	**7**	true	**9**	false
2	false	**5**	false	**8**	true	**10**	true
3	true	**6**	false				

8.4

1	raise	**5**	lost fluid and	**7**	boiled	**11**	incise
2	cloth		blood	**8**	foreign bodies	**12**	venom
3	maintain	**6**	antiseptic so-	**9**	skin or tissues	**13**	water
4	tourniquet		lution	**10**	tie off	**14**	limb
						15	antivenom

8.6

1 Did you eat at your aunt's?
2 The girl's medicine.
3 Can I get you a cup of tea?

4 He works at the butcher's.
5 There are a number of things.

8.7

1 attendances (l. 10/11, 21/22)
2 inappropriate (l. 11/12)
3 load (l. 15)
4 classified (l. 11)

5 unjustifiable (l. 21)
6 shortfalls (l. 2)
7 adequate (l. 20)
8 stretched (l. 16)

8.8

1 Aufrechterhaltung
2 künstliche Beatmung
3 entzogen
4 Bewusstlosigkeit
5 Herzstillstand
6 blockieren
7 Luftwege
8 Kiefer
9 ersticken
10 entfernen

11 Luftröhre
12 Klapse
13 Sauerstoffversorgung
14 aufblasen, mit Luft füllen
15 kippen
16 Nasenloch/Nasenflügel
17 kneifen
18 Halsschlagader
19 schwach
20 hin- und herbewegen

1 **a** a drink of beer
  b a measure for liquids
2 **a** female sibling
  b female charge nurse
3 **a** a male parent
  b title of respect for priest ('Father')
4 **a** to press between thumb and finger
  b to arrest
5 **a** to seize by the power of the law
  b to stop (cardiac arrest)

6 **a** to look after a patient
  b to suck milk from a woman's breast
7 **a** perspiration
  b an anxious state
8 **a** diaphragm (also 'Dutch cap')
  b a flat covering for the head
9 **a** a thick strong metal rope
  b a telegram
10 **a** having a large distance between opposite surfaces
  b stupid, slow to understand

1 United Kingdom
2 United Kingdom Central Council (for Nursing, Midwifery and Health Visiting)
3 Registered General Nurse
4 all correct
5 (Latin: ante meridiem) before noon
6 charge nurse
7 chronic obstructive airway disease
8 chronic heart failure
9 against medical advice
10 left ventricle failure
11 admission specimen urine
12 nasogastric tube
13 pulmonary embolism
14 per requestum
15 do not resuscitate
16 below-knee amputation
17 (Latin: ter in die) three times a day
18 senile dementia of Alzheimer's type
19 nausea, vomiting, diarrhoea
20 total parenteral nutrition
21 as tolerated
22 out of bed
23 as soon as possible
24 (Latin: quaque 2 hora) every two hours
25 checks
26 blood pressure and temperature
27 patient's
28 laboratory
29 bowel movement
30 passed urine

9.2 [Lat.] = kommt aus dem Lateinischen

1 Geburtsdatum
2 unbekannt
3 ausgeschlossen
4 Länge
5 Gewicht
6 Behandlung
7 Fraktur, Bruch
8 Bauch
9 Gelenk
10 Schmerzen im unteren Rücken

Unit 9

11 wie gewünscht
12 dünnflüssig (Diät)
13 direkt (Rezepte) [Lat. statim]
14 lokal
15 ambulant
16 Familienstand

17 jede zweite Nacht [Lat. alternis noctibus]
18 ausreichende Menge [Lat. quantum sufficit]
19 Poliklinik
20 plötzlicher Kindstod

9.4

1-d, **2**-f, **3**-h, **4**-j, **5**-b, **6**-l, **7**-i, **8**-m, **9**-c, **10**-g, **11**-a, **12**-k, **13**-e

9.5

1 worse
2 most cheerful
3 most comfortable
4 thinner
5 smallest

6 narrower
7 more careless
8 dirtier
9 busiest
10 most exciting

9.7

1 unzureichend
2 Anstieg
3 nicht in der Lage sein
4 Veränderung in
5 Stimmungsumschwung
6 Verschlechterung, Beeinträchtigung von
7 ungeeignet
8 vermindert

9 potential for risk
10 progress
11 cross/frustrate/counteract
12 limited
13 failure to
14 difficulty in
15 loss of

9.8

1 Impairment of mobility related to varicose veins.
2 Restricted joint movements related to inflamed joints/arthritis.
3 Feels depressed and is no longer able to cope.
4 Expressed anxiety at the involvement of the social services.
5 Cannot get up or walk unaided.

6 Separation anxiety arising from hospitalisation.
7 Possible infection through reduced resistance.
8 Propensity/inclination to fall.
9 Patient is unwilling to communicate.
10 Discuss patient's own perception of the problem.

1 before meals
2 alternate days/every other day
3 alternate hours
4 twice a day
5 twice a night
6 hour
7 hour of sleep
8 night
9 (Latin: post meridiem) after noon
10 every day
11 every hour
12 four times a day
13 every morning
14 every night

15 every other day
16 admission, discharge, transfer
17 bed rest
18 bathroom privileges
19 discontinue
20 do not intubate
21 diagnosis
22 history
23 not applicable
24 no complaints
25 nothing by mouth
26 prognosis
27 symptoms
28 year of birth

10.1

1-d, **2**-a, **3**-b, **4**-d, **5**-a, **6**-d, **7**-c, **8**-c, **9**-b

10.2

1 heel
2 calf
3 shin
4 buttock
5 forearm
6 elbow
7 upperarm
8 shoulder blade (scapula)
9 nape of the neck

10 back
11 loin
12 waist
13 thumb
14 index finger
15 middle finger
16 ring finger
17 little finger
18 wrist

10.3

1 instep
2 toes
3 ankle
4 knee
5 thigh

6 groin
7 abdomen
8 thorax/chest
9 axilla/armpit
10 elbow

11 hip
12 back of the
knee/popliteal
space
13 little toe/

5th toe
14 4th toe
15 3rd toe
16 2nd toe
17 big toe

Unit 10

10.4

1	heavy	**3**	severely	**6**	easily	**9**	remarkably
2	fully/completely	**4**	early	**7**	hardly	**10**	extensive
		5	badly	**8**	differently		

10.5

1 Rest in plaster is the only treatment required.
2 The senses of taste and smell are closely linked.
3 Chewed food first travels through the oesophagus.
4 The child's heart is beating irregularly/heartbeat is irregular.
5 He can hardly stand up.

10.6

1	diaphragm	**4**	kidneys	**7**	colon	**10**	thyroid
2	stomach	**5**	bladder	**8**	rectum	**11**	trachea
3	spleen	**6**	duodenum	**9**	larynx		

10.7

1 to improve
2 to encourage
3 to sterilize
4 to disinfect/decontaminate
5 to evaluate
6 to assess
7 to assist
8 to coordinate
9 to tune/gear to
10 to close off
11 to interrupt
12 to proceed/continue
13 to question/interview
14 to examine
15 to resuscitate
16 to support
17 to inject
18 to give up/abandon
19 to discontinue
20 to insert
21 to cope
22 to need
23 to express
24 to discuss
25 to ease/alleviate/relieve/soothe
26 to arrange
27 to result in
28 to estimate
29 to cause
30 to indicate

1	cranium	**10**	pubis	**21**	carpals	**33**	acromion
2	zygomatic bone	**11**	ischium	**22**	phalanges	**34**	olecranon
3	mandible	**12**	symphysis pubis	**23**	metacarpals	**35**	ilium
4	maxilla	**13**	femur	**24**	femur	**36**	coccyx
5	xiphoid process	**14**	clavicle	**25**	patella	**37**	lateral condyle
6	costal cartilage	**15**	scapula	**26**	tibia	**38**	medial condyle
7	vertebral column	**16**	sternum	**27**	fibula	**39**	lateral malleolus
8	ilium	**17**	ribs	**28**	tarsal	**40**	medial malleolus
9	sacrum	**18**	humerus	**29**	metatarsals	**41**	calcaneus
		19	ulna	**30**	phalanges		
		20	radius	**31**	parietal (bone)		
				32	occipital bone		

10.9

1	fibula	**5**	uterus	**9**	ligament	**13**	tongue
2	joint	**6**	thyroid	**10**	spleen	**14**	ureter
3	pancreas	**7**	bronchiole	**11**	prostate	**15**	finishing point
4	foreskin	**8**	tonsil	**12**	peritoneum		

1-b, **2**-d, **3**-c, **4**-a, **5**-b, **6**-c, **7**-b, **8**-c, **9**-d

11.2

1-B, **2**-C, **3**-A, **4**-g, **5**-i, **6**-h, **7**-k, **8**-I, **9**-d, **10**-e, **11**-f, **12**-m, **13**-j

11.4

1	to expectorate	**7**	to understand
2	to fell queasy/sick – to vomit	**8**	to leave the bed – to collapse – to regain conscience
3	to omit	**9**	to gain weight – to reduce weight
4	to button	**10**	to be very upset
5	to bear it	**11**	to improve
6	to irritate		

11.5

1 Who are your next of kin?/significant others?
2 How do you feel about your situation/your disease?
3 Can you describe your pain?/Where does it hurt?/Since when does it hurt?
4 Is there anything I can help you with?/Is there anything I can do for you?
5 How did you cope at home?

11.6

1 will be – survives
2 gets – will bring
3 have arrived –
4 go – will not sleep
5 will be discharged – has healed
6 if
7 when
8 If
9 We'll talk about your treatment as soon as we have received the last result of the x-ray.
10 Before you take the job you must have a medical check-up.

11.7

1 * Informiere den Patienten darüber, was ihn vor und nach der Operation erwartet, z.B. über Drainagen, Katheter, Atemübungen, usw.
   * Ermittle, ob und welche Ängste der Patient möglicherweise hat, und bespreche diese mit ihm
2 * Überprüfe bei jedem Lagewechsel die Unversehrtheit des Hautzustandes
   * Entwerfe einen Lagerungsplan und führe einen zweistündlichen Lagewechsel durch
3 * Encourage the patient to express feelings of anxiety, fear of mutilation or of refusal
   * Encourage the patient to look at and touch her body/her scars
4 * Provide communication aids (e.g. blackboards, pictures)
   * Keep calm and supporting, give the patient enough time to speak and answer

11.8

1 true
2 false
3 true
4 false
5 true

1	Homeopathy	**4**	Healing	**7**	Alternative	**10**	Reflexology
2	Massage	**5**	Counselling	**8**	Psychotherapy	**11**	Osteopathy
3	Hypnotherapy	**6**	Acupuncture	**9**	Herbalism		